www.harcourt-internatic

Bringing you products from all Harcourt Health Sciences companies including Baillière Tindall, Churchill Livingstone, Mosby and W.B. Saunders

▶ **Browse** for latest information on new books, journals and electronic products

▶ **Search** for information on over 20 000 published titles with full product information including tables of contents and sample chapters

▶ **Keep up to date** with our extensive publishing programme in your field by registering with eAlert or requesting postal updates

▶ **Secure online ordering** with prompt delivery, as well as full contact details to order by phone, fax or post

▶ **News** of special features and promotions

If you are based in the following countries, please visit the country-specific site to receive full details of product availability and local ordering information

USA: www.harcourthealth.com

Canada: www.harcourtcanada.com

Australia: www.harcourt.com.au

Baillière Tindall   CHURCHILL LIVINGSTONE   Mosby   W.B. SAUNDERS

Pharmaceutical and Medicines
Information Management

Commissioning Editor: Timothy Horne
Project Development Manager: Lynn Watt
Project Manager: Nancy Arnott
Design direction: Judith Wright

PHARMACEUTICAL AND MEDICINES INFORMATION MANAGEMENT
Principles and Practice

Edited by

Andrew S. Robson
GlaxoSmithKline Pharmaceuticals
Harlow, Essex, UK

David Bawden
Department of Information Science
City University, London, UK

Alan Judd
Consultant Medicines Information Pharmacist
Leeds, UK

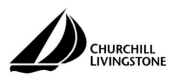

CHURCHILL
LIVINGSTONE

EDINBURGH LONDON NEW YORK PHILADELPHIA ST LOUIS SYDNEY TORONTO 2001

CHURCHILL LIVINGSTONE
An imprint of Harcourt Publishers Limited

© Harcourt Publishers Limited 2001

◢ is a registered trademark of Harcourt Publishers Limited

The right of Andrew S. Robson, David Bawden and Alan Judd to be identified as editor
of this work has been asserted by them in accordance with the Copyright, Designs and
Patents Act 1988

First published 2001

ISBN 0-443-06401-6

British Library Cataloguing in Publication Data
A catalogue record for this book is available from the British Library

Library of Congress Cataloging in Publication Data
A catalog record for this book is available from the Library of Congress

Note
Medical knowledge is constantly changing. As new information becomes available,
changes in treatment, procedures, equipment and the use of drugs become necessary.
The editor and the publishers have taken care to ensure that the information given in
this text is accurate and up to date. However, readers are strongly advised to confirm
that the information, especially with regard to drug usage, complies with the latest
legislation and standards of practice.

The
Publisher's
policy is to use
**paper manufactured
from sustainable forests**

Printed in China

Contents

Preface

Many of today's medicines are the results of extensive research programmes that produce huge volumes of data and information. Then, once a medicine is available on the market, ever more experience and information about its efficacy and safety accumulate. So much information, published and unpublished, is available about modern medicines that it is almost impossible for individuals to cope with the overload.

Too often in this 'Information Age' we assume that advances in computer technology will meet all of our information needs. Too infrequently is consideration given to the skills involved in managing information and knowledge. There are many publications about the use of computer systems in medicine and in the pharmaceutical industry, yet there are few books devoted to the range of skills, tools and knowledge needed to find, evaluate and communicate information about medicines. This book seeks to fill that gap.

The following chapters describe information management roles in hospitals and in the pharmaceutical industry: they cover legal and ethical issues and also consider professional development and the management of information services.

Condensing this subject matter into a manageable package is not an easy task. Fortunately we have been able to call upon expert contributors; all of whom have extensive practical experience and many have lectured on the MSc/Diploma course in Pharmaceutical Information Management at City University London. The syllabus of this course, which was established in 1997, provided us with a structure. The book's contents include the main subject areas covered by the course, with additional reference material and reading lists.

This is not intended to be solely an academic textbook. It is a practical handbook, guiding the reader in finding information about medicines and in evaluating and interpreting that information. Anybody who is interested in modern medicines or in the skills involved in finding and using information about medicines and related subjects will find something of use to them in the following pages.

In dealing with such a rapidly developing field as information management, it is inevitable that some changes will have occurred by the time this book is published. One development that occurred just as the book was being finalized was a change in terminology for UK hospital information pharmacists. As explained in Chapter 8, the term 'Medicines Information' is replacing 'Drug Information'. Since 'Drug Information' has been used for many years and is still the term used in the USA and elsewhere, we decided to retain it rather than make last-minute alterations to the page proofs. Readers should be aware, however, that the preferred term in the UK is 'Medicines Information'.

Andrew S. Robson
David Bawden
Alan Judd

Acknowledgements

We wish to thank everybody who has been involved in the development and production of this book. In particular we are grateful to all the contributors, who agreed so willingly to give of their time and to share their expertise. We are also very grateful to the publisher, Harcourt Health Sciences, for responding so positively to our initial proposals and for patiently seeing the project through. Special thanks are due to Timothy Horne, Sarah Keer-Keer and Lynn Watt.

Andrew S. Robson
David Bawden
Alan Judd

Contributors

David Bawden BSc, MSc, PhD
Course Director
Department of Information Science
City University
Northampton Square
London

Collette Beglin BSc, Dip Reg Affairs, MBIRA
Unicus Regulatory Services Ltd
Foxtwist Farm
New Mill Road
Finchampstead
Berkshire

Geraldine Boyce PhD
Published Information
GlaxoSmithKline
New Frontiers Science Park
Harlow
Essex

Sandy Chalmers BSc, MIInfSc
Data Privacy Advisor
European Regulatory Affairs
GlaxoSmithKline
Greenford Rd
Greenford, Middlesex

Janet E. Davies BPharm, MRPharmS, MIInfSc
Director of Medical Services
Bristol-Myers Squibb Pharmaceuticals
141–149 Staines Road
Hounslow
Middlesex

Secretary and Past President, AIOPI (Association of Information Officers in the Pharmaceutical Industry)

Elisabeth Goodman BSc, MSc, MIInfSci
Knowledge Tools
GlaxoSmithKline
Ware
Hertfordshire

Neil Gow BSc
Regulatory Information Management Specialist
British Biotech Pharmaceuticals
Oxford

Elena Grant B.Pharm, MSc, MCPP, MRPharmS
Regional Medicines Information Pharmacist
West Midlands Medicines Information Pharmacist
Good Hope Hospital NHS Trust
Sutton Coldfield
West Midlands

David E. Hands BPharm, FRPharmS, DMS
Formerly Principal Pharmacist
South and West Drug Information Service (Southampton)
Southampton General Hospital
Southampton

Shapour Hariri BSc, PhD
Business Development Manager
Diligenti Ltd
303 Ballards Lane
London

Caroline M. Holden BTech (Hons), DipInfSc, MIInfSc
eHealthcare Consultant
eMed-Media
St Peter's Institute
Windmill Street
Macclesfield

Alan Judd BSc Pharm, MSc, PhD, MRPharmS
Consultant Medicines Information Pharmacist
Formerly Director
Regional Drug and Poisons Information Service
Leeds

Frank N. Leach BPharm, MSc, PhD, MRPharms
North West Regional Drug Information Service
St Mary's Hospital
Manchester

Sharon Leighton BSc, PhD
Head of Medical Information & Drug Safety
AstraZeneca UK Ltd
Horizon Place
600 Capability Green
Luton, Bedfordshire

Past President, AIOPI (Association of Information Officers in the Pharmaceutical Industry)

Debbie Morrison MA(Cantab)
Information Management
GlaxoSmithKline
New Frontiers Science Park
Harlow
Essex

Charles Oppenheim BSc, PhD, DipInfSc, CertEd, FIInfSc, FLA, FRSA, AUMIST
Professor of Information Science
Loughborough University
Loughborough
Leicestershire

Elizabeth Orna PhD, FIInfSc
Information Consultant
Orna Information and Editorial Consultancy
55 Telegraph Lane East
Norwich
Norfolk

Jennifer L. Riggins PharmD
Eli Lilly and Company
Lilly Corporate Center
Indianapolis, IN
USA

Lyn Robinson BSc, MSc
Visiting Scholar
City University
Northampton Square
London

Andrew S. Robson BSc, MSc
Head, Global Medical Information
GlaxoSmithKline
New Frontiers Science Park South
Third Avenue
Harlow
Essex

Ian Rowlands BSc, MSc, PhD
Course Director
Department of Information Science
City University
Northampton Square
London

Heather Simmonds BSc
Director
Prescription Medicines Code of Practice Authority
12 Whitehall
London

Lesley West PhD
Director
CERES West Ltd
Teddington
London

Jane Whittall BSc, MSc, MIInfSci
Head
Published Information, Information Management
GlaxoSmithKline
New Frontiers Science Park
Harlow
Essex

Chapter 1

Introduction

Andrew S Robson and David Bawden

The aim of this book is to describe and provide guidance on the knowledge and skills involved in finding, interpreting and communicating information about medicines. The main focus is on the roles and activities of staff in pharmaceutical companies and in hospital pharmacies who provide information services about medicines for human use (including compounds in development). Different services have different titles such as 'drug information', 'medical information', 'research/scientific information' and so on. 'Pharmaceutical and medicines information' was chosen for the book's title as an umbrella term to refer to these different types of information services.

The book should also be of value to those involved in dealing with pharmaceutical information in other environments, such as publishing, medical writing, database production, clinical trials organization, promotional activities and consultancy.

Reliable and usable information is as much a part of the medicines 'package' as the physical formulation. Healthcare professionals, including physicians, pharmacists and nurses must have up-to-date, accurate information and knowledge about medicines in order to use them effectively and safely. Pharmacists in hospital drug information centres play an essential role in providing such information. Information departments in pharmaceutical companies also play a key role, as companies have uniquely comprehensive collections of information about the medicines that they develop and market.

Within companies, effective management of information is also crucial in research and development, in registration of medicines and in supporting marketing and sales activities. Not for nothing is the pharmaceutical industry known as the 'information intensive' industry par excellence, arguably the first example of the truly knowledge-based industry.

The drug information pharmacists and industry staff who provide these services are highly skilled in finding information, in analysing and evaluating it and in communicating it in a form that meets the needs of their customers. They are also knowledgeable about the medicines and compounds with which they deal. In addition, they are skilled in the use of information technology, and often play a part in the development of new electronic information systems.

The importance of library and information services in patient care has been documented in numerous studies (e.g. Bond et al 1999, King 1987, Marshall 1992, Veenstra 1992). However, in many discussions on the management of information, emphasis is given to information technology (IT) rather than to the importance of knowledge about the subject area and the skills needed to interpret information. IT is certainly important and provides valuable tools to help store, retrieve, process and transmit information. However, information technology does not equate to information management. Effective information management—and knowledge management perhaps more so—requires human skills and expertise.

This book aims to change the emphasis. While it describes IT tools and information management processes that are of value in pharmaceutical information management, it focuses on the skills that are needed to provide high quality information services.

Hospital-based drug information centres were first established in the USA in the early 1960s (Amerson & Wallingford 1983). They were soon also established in the UK (see Chapter 8) and other countries. Information departments in the pharmaceutical industry have existed for at least as long (see, for example, Haygarth-Jackson 1977, 1987). Over the years, the numbers of drug information centres and industry information departments have increased and their roles have expanded. The prediction of future trends is as difficult for pharmaceutical information provision as in any other aspect of professional life (Bawden 1997, 1998), but it seems clear that this expansion and diversification of roles will continue. The need for a sound basic education and for relevant and effective continuing professional development for pharmaceutical information professionals is therefore more important than ever.

Entrants to pharmaceutical information work come with diverse backgrounds, combining, in varied proportions, formal qualifications and practical experience in the background sciences and in library/information science and IT. Although some academic institutions in the UK and in Continental Europe offer short courses, and specialist modules within broader courses, in pharmaceutical information, prior to 1997 there was no specialist academic course devoted to this area.

Recognizing the need for such a specialist course, a combined group of academics and experienced pharmaceutical information professionals in the UK established a postgraduate MSc/Diploma in Pharmaceutical Information Management at City University London in 1997. The course was set up in association with, and continues to be supported by, AIOPI (the Association of Information Officers in the Pharmaceutical Industry) and the UK DIPG (Drug Information Pharmacists Group). The syllabus built upon experience gained with programmes of practical information skills training developed by AIOPI and the DIPG. It also benefited from City University London's long experience with postgraduate courses in information science and information technology, including pharmaceutical information specialisms.

This book has developed together with the MSc/Diploma course. Although it is based to a large extent on the syllabus of that course, it is intended as a reference work in its own right. The editors and authors hope that it will be of interest and value to a wide readership. There are few other up-to-date books that cover the subjects that appear in the following chapters and none, so far as we are aware, which deal with the full range of topics included here; nor are we aware of any written in collaboration between experts from academia, hospital pharmacy and the pharmaceutical industry.

Pharmaceutical information is now very much a multinational concern, not least because of factors such as the increasing globalization of large pharmaceutical companies and their branded products, and the increasingly transnational scope of regulation. Although the book is written mainly by UK-based contributors, the scope is far from parochial. Just as the MSc course attracts an international group of students, so we believe that this book will be of value to an international audience.

The chapters cover a number of themes relevant to information services about medicines.

- Chapters 2 and 3 review the 'tools of the trade'—information sources and information technology. Chapter 4 then describes some of the main concepts and issues in the management of information and knowledge.

- The next three chapters cover key skills. Chapter 5 describes a logical process for dealing with enquiries and providing information. Chapter 6 describes the principles involved in analysing and evaluating evidence about the clinical use of medicines. Chapter 7 discusses the skills needed in managing an information service.

- Chapters 8 to 15 describe roles and specific skills involved in pharmaceutical information management. Included are hospital-based drug information services (Chapter 8) and information management roles in the pharmaceutical industry (Chapters 9 to 15), though material in these latter chapters is relevant in a wider context.

- Chapters 16 to 18 deal with legal, ethical and related issues concerning information services, with emphasis on the issues in dealing with information on medicines.

■ Chapter 19 discusses careers and professional development in pharmaceutical information services.

It is not necessary to read the chapters in sequence. Each has been written to stand on its own. Although this implies some overlap of content, albeit from a different perspective, we regard this as a benefit for the reader.

With the continuing rapid growth in information about drugs and other therapies, and the increasing significance of the internet for provision of both professional and public information, information services in hospitals and in the pharmaceutical industry have a vital role to play in ensuring that medicines are used effectively and safely. This book will help providers of information services to further their knowledge and professional skills. It is hoped that it will also help them to develop their careers and to demonstrate the value that their services provide, thereby improving the image and standing of the information professions in the pharmaceutical environment.

In dealing with such a rapidly developing field as information management, it is inevitable that some changes will have occurred by the time this book is published. One development that occurred as the book was being finalized was a change in terminology for UK hospital information pharmacists. As explained in the preface, in Chapter 8 the term 'Medicines Information' is replacing 'Drug Information'. Since 'Drug Information' has been used for many years and is still the term used in the USA and elsewhere, we have decided to retain it rather than make last-minute alterations to the page proofs. Readers should be aware, however, that the preferred term in the UK is 'Medicines Information'.

References

Amerson A B, Wallingford D M 1983 Twenty years' experience with drug information centers. American Journal of Hospital Pharmacy 40: 1172–1178

Bawden D 1997 The nature of prediction and the information future: Arthur C Clarke's Odyssey vision. Aslib Proceedings 49(3): 57–60

Bawden D 1998 Information futures: literacy, overload or feudalism? Elizabeth Kenny memorial lecture, given at the 25th Annual Conference of AIOPI, Eastbourne, 6 July

Bond C A, Raehl C L, Franke T 1999 Clinical pharmacy services and hospital mortality rates. Pharmacotherapy 19(5): 556–564

Haygarth-Jackson A R 1997 Library and technical information services – ICI Pharmaceuticals Division. Aslib Proceedings 29(1): 337–347

Haygarth-Jackson A R 1987 Pharmaceuticals – an information-based industry. Aslib Proceedings 39(3): 75–86.

King D N 1987 The contribution of hospital library information services to critical care: a study in eight hospitals. Bulletin of the Medical Library Association 75(4): 291–301

Marshall J G 1992 The impact of the hospital library on clinical decision making: the Rochester study. Bulletin of the Medical Library Association 80(2): 169–178

Veenstra R J 1992 Clinical medical librarian impact on patient care: a one-year analysis. Bulletin of the Medical Library Association 80(1): 19–22

Chapter 2

Information sources

David Bawden and Lyn Robinson

Introduction

The information sources available to support the discovery, development and effective use of medicines are numerous, varied and rapidly changing. In this chapter, we will make no attempt at an exhaustive listing of useful resources; rather we will give a general overview of the kinds of resources available, with some examples.

A detailed review and discussion of a wide variety of pharmaceutical sources, though inevitably rather dated, is given by Pickering (1990). Morton & Godbolt (1992) cover sources in the medical area. A more recent account from the perspective of the pharmacist is given by Malone et al (1996).

One point which may be emphasized at the outset is that details of useful resources are now most readily gained from the internet, where all major publishers, database producers and other information providers give updated information on their products.

Categorization of information resources

There are four general ways in which information resources may be categorized:

- by subject
- by format
- by location
- by type of material.

Subject categorization

A breakdown by subject is not the most useful way of dealing with the topic, since many resources cover multiple subjects, leading to duplication and repetition. However, it is worth noting at this point the breadth of subjects which are relevant to pharmaceutical information in the broadest sense. While it is possible to define a core set of subjects of obvious relevance—pharmacology, pharmacy, aspects of chemistry, and of human and veterinary medicine, for example—the breadth of the scientific disciplines contributing to modern pharmaceutical research, and the equivalent breadth of subjects and disciplines involved in the marketing of medicines, and in the provision of advice as to their best use, makes it well-nigh impossible to set clear boundaries around the subjects which may be relevant.

An illustration of the breadth of scope, and the diversity, of information sources which may need to be accessed is given by the kinds of sources required for the pharmaceutical competitive intelligence function (Bawden 1998, Krol et al 1996):

- commercial databases (of varied kinds)
- patent documents and associated literature
- trade and industry periodicals
- trade and association reports
- newswires
- national newspaper articles
- press releases with company news
- press releases concerning scientific or medical developments
- articles and interviews in 'general' magazines
- articles in 'local' newspapers and magazines (relating to local companies)
- scientific and medical primary literature
- meetings abstracts (scientific and medical)
- meetings and seminar 'hand-outs'
- calls for proposals for research grants
- announcements of grants and similar funding
- company quarterly and annual reports
- other company publications (e.g. prospectuses)
- in-house company magazines
- product brochures
- company filings and accounts
- reports of court cases
- financial and industry analysts' reports
- Freedom of Information Act documents (USA only)
- consultancy reports
- directories
- recruitment advertisments
- business school case studies.

While all of these may be described as 'published', some are clearly in the area of 'grey' literature, beyond what would normally be handled by a library/information service.

Format categorization

The second form of framework is one based on format of information: printed book, online bibliographic database, web page etc. While this is a necessary element of information to know for a resource, it is not very useful as a primary framework; for one thing, some resources exist in several forms—e.g. Index Medicus/Medline exists as print, online, CD-ROM—leading to duplication.

It is, however, worth noting the variety of formats in which pharmaceutical information is provided; the general trend has been towards new formats being added to, rather than entirely supplanting, previous formats. Although there has been a steady move towards provision of a greater proportion of information in digital form, print-on-paper is still of considerable significance. Similarly, despite the increasing value of the internet for pharmaceutical information, as with other professional areas, it is far from the case that this now provides *all* important information. Internet sites with relevance to pharmaceuticals, as for healthcare generally, are numerous, diverse, and rapidly changing—see, for example, Wood (2000)—so that providing a comprehensive list is not feasible. The best starting point for an examination of this area are the subject gateways described elsewhere in this chapter.

The 'traditional' online host systems are still an important means of access to both bibliographic and factual/numeric sources: for pharmaceuticals, Dialog, Datastar and STN provide access to the key online databases. Access and interfaces to these host systems have been considerably changed under the influence of graphical interfaces generally, and the internet in particular; see Large et al (1999) for a good overview.

CD-ROM, though no longer regarded as the medium of the future, retains a niche, particularly for collections of material which do not require frequent updating; annual compendia for example.

Finally, the continuing importance of the human expert should be noted; individual contacts are still important in a digital age.

Location categorization

The third form of categorization divides resources according to location, e.g. country of origin. There is some justification for this in the case of legislative and regulatory aspects, which may well differ from country to country, but it is not overall a particularly helpful approach. This is particularly so when a good deal of information is networked, and it is largely irrelevant to know, and may be impossible to determine, the geographical location of a particular resource.

However, it is worth mentioning one significant distinction of this kind, and that is the distinction between internal and external information sources: *internal* sources are those created and maintained within an organization, generally including unpublished and proprietary information; *external* sources are publicly available resources. This chapter is largely devoted to external sources of pharmaceutical information, but at this point it is worth considering the value of the internal source.

Internal files

These files are generally regarded as falling into two main categories: those holding chemical, biological or clinical data, generally produced by, or of close relevance to, the organization's own research and development, and those holding files of literature references, selected for their relevance to the organization's activities.

Internal files may also hold specific forms of information: media reports about an organization, for example, or competitor intelligence, or internal reports and other documentation. A newer form of internal resource is the 'know how' database, a collection of in-house expertise, whether represented by a link to the individual—an 'expertise index'—or by some explicit account of in-house knowledge.

Internal databanks are generally built around database management systems, often with a specific chemical structure-handling capability. Links are often provided to information processing systems, to add capabilities such as structure-property correlation, molecular modelling, statistical analysis, and graphical display and tabulation.

Internal literature databases, created and operated by research or commercial organizations, are generally referred to as 'in-house' databases. They may be very specifically subject-oriented (most obviously towards a company's own products) and employ specific criteria for coverage, with specific indexing languages and policies. In-house files of this sort have been found to be of value in several studies particularly because of their wide coverage of material which may not be found in other sources (see, for example Bawden & Brock 1982) and more generally because they provide high levels of recall and precision in retrieval of biomedical material (see, for example Gretz & Thomas 1995, Robinson et al 2000, Sodha & van Amelsvoort 1994).

'Type' categorization

This leaves the fourth type of framework, in which resources are initially categorized according to their type, in general terms. The most generally useful categorization is an adaptation of a 'traditional' library/information framework, based on structure of literature, particularly scientific literature (Robinson 2000a). Resources are divided into primary, secondary, tertiary, and (sometimes) quaternary categories, essentially according to their distance along the communication chain from the original 'raw' information. A particularly clear and full description is given by Grogan (1970). Adaptation is necessary because this model was derived for a system of publication based purely on printed products. Limited modification coped with the inclusion of computerized sources, e.g. machine-readable abstracting and indexing services, but the arrival of the new forms of information product on the internet requires the model to be extended further. Nonetheless it is noteworthy that this relatively elderly model, when appropriately modified, still serves very well in helping to clarify the allegedly chaotic system of (largely networked) information of the present time.

Under this system, resources are categorized as follows:

- Primary: the original information, in whatever form it takes
- Secondary: 'worked over' knowledge, which organizes the primary material in some way
- Tertiary: rather diverse sources, which aid the use of resources at other levels; typically they do not provide substantive 'subject' information in themselves
- Quaternary: give access to resource listings at a high level, not usually subject specific.

Primary and secondary resources are subject specific by this definition, tertiary may or may not be. Quaternary are not usually subject specific.

There is a further, *zeroth* order, of information; the 'raw' data which comes from laboratory instruments: however, although this can now be readily captured, stored and transmitted elsewhere, it is not truly an information resource until it has been organized and described so as to be understandable in 'public use', at which stage it can be regarded as primary information. However, this form of information, most commonly now handled in laboratory instrument management systems (LIMS), is an important source of internal information for regulatory purposes.

Examples of the other four categories follow.

Primary

- journal articles, pre-prints (paper and electronic)
- reports
- data tabulations
- laboratory notebooks
- diaries
- memoranda, letters, email messages, postings to newsgroups
- conference proceedings
- theses, dissertations
- patents
- standards
- regulations and legislation
- trade and product information, technical manuals
- course notes, interactive training materials, syllabi
- company reports, financial data
- organizations' and individuals' homepages.

Secondary

- reviews and summaries of progress
- indexing and abstracting services
- data compilations, databanks
- monographs, textbooks, treatises
- reference works, encyclopaedias, handbooks, data tables
- dictionaries, thesauri, classification schemes, glossaries.

Monographs and textbooks still play an important role for reference information. Although a few major texts are becoming available in digital form, the Oxford Textbook of Medicine being a well-known example, print is still a convenient medium for this sort of compendium. Other examples of well-known textbooks, from many available, are:

- Goodman and Gilman's Pharmacological Basis of Therapeutics (McGraw-Hill, 9th edn, 1996)
- Meyler's Side Effects of Drugs (Elsevier, annual editions)
- Stockley's Drug Interactions (Blackwell, 3rd edn, 1996)
- Ganong's Review of Medical Physiology (Prentice Hall, 16th edn, 1993).

Other kinds of secondary sources of importance to drug information include:

- handbooks, e.g. Merck Index and Handbook of Pharmaceutical Excipients (Pharmaceutical Press, 3rd edn, 2000)
- encyclopaedias, e.g. Encyclopedia of Controlled Drug Delivery (Wiley, 1999)
- dictionaries, e.g. Dictionary of Antibiotics and related substances (CRC Press, 1997) and Dorland's Illustrated Medical Dictionary (WB Saunders, 29th edn, 2000)
- thesauri, e.g. UK DIPG's Pharmline Thesaurus.

Again, these tools are still often produced in print form for convenient and immediate look-up, commonly running into several editions, though electronic versions are appearing.

Pharmaceutical material appears in many *tertiary sources*. Often, however, it is subsumed within a resource dealing with a more general discipline, e.g. healthcare, or a specific aspect, e.g. antibiotics, rather than being simply denoted as pharmaceutical. As with other kinds of resources, tertiary pharmaceutical resources exist in a variety of formats, with paper generally being complemented by, or replaced by, digital sources.

Examples are directories of relevant health professionals, British examples being the Medical Directory and Medical Register for doctors and the Annual Register of Pharmaceutical Chemists for pharmacists.

A new form of tertiary resource is the internet subject gateway or virtual library (Robinson & Bawden 1999). Several examples of this exist for pharmaceuticals, in a variety of forms from the simple to the complex. The simpler sort is exemplified by the worldwide web Virtual Library for Pharmacy (www.cpb.uokhsc.edu/pharmacy/pharmint.html), a categorized list of relevant internet resources. This is taken a step further in the so-called 'quality gateways', which choose sites to be listed by a careful assessment of quality; an example is the OMNI healthcare internet gateway (www.omni.ac.uk). The more complex forms of gateway are exemplified by Pharmweb, a UK site, (www.pharmweb.net) and a US equivalent PharmInfoNet (pharminfo.net). Both offer lists of relevant resources, but also data compilations, news items, and specialised discussion groups.

Quaternary resources, useful as an initial entry into sources in an unfamiliar area, or as part of comprehensive review, are less likely to be pharmaceutically specific than to cover a wider subject area. Examples are the collections of online library catalogues provided by the UK NISS information gateway (www.niss.ac.uk), and various internet 'lists of lists', such as the Magellan Internet directory (magellan.excite.com) and the Pinakes list of subject gateways (www.hw.ac.uk/libWWW/irn/pinakes/pinakes.html).

Quaternary resources are likely to be used only occasionally, as the need arises, but tertiary, secondary and primary resources are likely to figure in lists of 'favourite sources', maintained explicitly or implicitly by most experienced pharmaceutical information workers. As an example, a selective list of printed sources is shown in Box 2.3 (this list is based on a personal selection of sources provided by Andrew Robson for the City University course, and slightly modified by the chapter authors). It is an example of the continuing value of the printed monograph and reference book, in a supposedly digital age.

A similar selective list, this time including digital sources, is the list of recommended sources produced by the UK Drug Information Pharmacists Group, in their Drug

Box 2.3 *Selective list of printed medical information sources*

Dictionaries
Butterworth's Medical Dictionary, Critchley M, ed. London:Butterworth; 1998
Dorland's Illustrated Medical Dictionary 29th edn, Anderson DM, ed. Philadelphia: WB Saunders, 2000

Drug names and synonyms
Index Nominum, International Drug Directory 16th edn, Swiss Pharmaceutical Society, Stuttgart: Medpharm Scientific Publishers; 1995
Organic-chemical Drugs and their Synonyms 7th edn, Negwer M, Berlin: Akademy Verlag; 1994

Drug guides and data sources
ABPI Compendium of Data Sheets and Summaries of Product Characteristics Association of the British Pharmaceutical Industry London: Datapharm Publications, every 15 months
British National Formulary, London: British Medical Association; Royal Pharmaceutical Society of Great Britain, twice yearly
MIMS, Monthly Index of Medical Specialities, London: Haymarket Publishing
Physicians' Desk Reference, Montvale, NJ: Medical Economics Company, annual
Martindale, the Extra Pharmacopoeia 31st edn, Reynolds J E F ed. London: Pharmaceutical Press; 1996
Therapeutic Drugs, Dollery C ed. Edinburgh: Churchill Livingstone; 1991

Textbooks
Goodman and Gilman's Pharmaceutical Basis of Therapeutics 9th edn, Hardman J G et al eds. New York: McGraw Hill; 1996.
Pharmacology 3rd edn, Rang H P et al, Edinburgh: Churchill Livingstone; 1995
Textbook of Pharmaceutical Medicine, Griffin J P et al eds. Belfast: Queens University of Belfast; 1993
Oxford Textbook of Medicine 3rd edn, Weatherall D J et al eds. Oxford: Oxford Medical Publications; 1996
Davidson's Principles and Practice of Medicine 17th edn, Edwards C R W, Bouchier I A D eds. Edinburgh: Churchill Livingstone; 1995
Review of Medical Physiology 16th edn, Ganong W F ed. East Norwalk: Lange; 1993

Drug safety
Meyler's Side Effects of Drugs 13th edn, Dukes M N G ed. Amsterdam: Elsevier; 1996
Side Effects of Drugs Annual, Vol. 22 Aronson J K, ed. Amsterdam: Elsevier; 1999
Drug Interactions, 3rd edn, Stockley I H, Oxford: Blackwell; 1996
Detection of New Adverse Drug Reactions 4th edn, Stephens M D B et al eds. London: MacMillan; 1998

Evidence–based practice
Evidence-based Medicine, How to Practise and Teach EBM, Sackett D L et al eds. Edinburgh: Churchill Livingstone; 1997
How to Read a Paper, the Basics of evidence-based Medicine, Greenhalgh T, London: BMJ Publishing Group; 1997
Medical Statistics, a Commonsense Approach, Campbell M J, Machin D eds. Chichester: John Wiley; 1997
The Pocket Guide to Critical Appraisal, Crombie I K, London: BMJ Publishing Group; 1996

Directories
Medical Directory, London: FT Healthcare, annual
Medical Register, Cambridge: General Medical Council/ Cambridge University Press, annual
Annual Register of Pharmaceutical Chemists, London: Royal Pharmaceutical Society of Great Britain

Information Manual. A summary of this annotated list is given in Box 2.4. Note the importance attached to organizations and individual expertise, in this case limited to UK examples.

A newer equivalent of this is the set of personally preferred internet sites, usually kept as individual or group 'favourites' or bookmarks. The large number and dynamic nature of

Box 2.4 *DIPG recommended sources*

Reference Sources
- Martindale, The Extra Pharmacopoeia
- Goodman and Gilman's Pharmacological Basis of Therapeutics
- Applied Therapeutics—The clinical use of drugs
- Dollery's Therapeutic Drugs
- Meyler's Side Effects of Drugs
- Side Effects of Drugs Annual
- ABPI Data Sheet Compendium
- British National Formulary
- American Society of Hospital Pharmacists drug information monographs
- Drugdex (full-text database)
- Patient Information leaflet compendium (ABPI)

Secondary Services
- Inpharma
- Clin-Alert
- International Pharmaceutical Abstracts
- Pharm-Line
- Iowa Drug Information Service
- Medline
- Excerpta Medica
- Review journals, especially *Drugs* and *Clinical Pharmacokinetics*

Primary Sources
- Scientific journals, particularly *British Medical Journal, Lancet, Journal of the American Medical Association* and *New England Journal of Medicine*
- Manufacturer's promotional material

Organizations
- Royal Pharmaceutical Society
- National Pharmaceutical Association
- Institute for the Study of Drug Dependence
- Release (for drug abuse)
- Poisons information service
- Committee on Safety of Medicines
- Employment Medical Advisory Service (part of Health and Safety Executive)
- Malaria Reference Laboratory
- National Drug Information Specialist Advisory and Information Services
- Pharmaceutical companies, and other manufacturing industry
- University and civic libraries
- Schools of pharmacy

internet sites of potential relevance to pharmaceutical information means that any attempt to provide a complete listing is doomed to failure, but a set of useful sites, to exemplify the variety available, is given in Box 2.5.

Evaluating and choosing sources

Given the range and diversity of potentially useful sources outlined above, it will be evident that one important task for the pharmaceutical information specialist will be the evaluation and selection of sources; for their own use, for recommendation to others. It is sometimes argued that, with the increased importance of digital as against printed sources, implying a need to obtain access to, rather than to acquire, resources, evaluation is less important, since we can simply 'use everything we have access to'. This is far from the truth; the plethora of available sources gives great potential for time-wasting, at best, and use of erroneous or sub-standard information, at worst, if careful evaluation is not performed.

Box 2.5 *Selective list of examples of relevant internet sites*

General gateways and search engines
SearchEngineWatch www.searchenginewatch.com
Pinakes list of subject gateways www.hw.ac.uk/libWWW/irn/pinakes/pinakes.html
BUBL subject gateway www.bubl.ac.uk
Omni healthcare gateway www.omni.ac.uk
Reuters Health eLine www.reutershealth.com
NHS Direct www.nhsdirect.nhs.uk

Subject specific gateways and portals
World Wide Web Virtual Library for Pharmacy www.cpb.uokhsc.edu/pharmacy/pharmit.html
Pharmweb www.pharmweb.net
PharmInfoNet pharminfo.com
MedicineNet www.medicinenet.com

Drug indexes and online pharmacies
RxList Internet Drug Index www.rxlist.com
Electronic Medicines Compendium www.emc.vhn.net
Allcures.com www.allcures.com
Pharmacy 2U www.pharmacy2u.co.uk

Associations
Association of the British Pharmaceutical Industry www.abpi.org.uk
Association of Information Officers in the Pharmaceutical Industry www.aiopi.org.uk
UK Drug Information Pharmacists Group www.ukdipg.org.uk
World Health Organization www.who.int

Regulatory Authorities
US FDA www.fda.gov
Medicines Control Agency (UK) www.open.gov.uk/mca
Committee on Safety of Medicines (UK) www.open.gov.uk/mca/csmhome.htm
European Medicinal Evaluation Agency www.emea.eu.int
National Institute for Clinical Excellence (UK) www.nice.org.uk/index.htm

Pharmaceutical Companies
consult the lists provided by sources such as PharmWeb *and* PharmInfoNet

Information providers
United States Pharmacopoeia www.usp.org
Adis www.adis.com
PJB Publications www.pjbpubs.co.uk
National Library of Medicine www.nlm.nih.gov
Chemical Abstracts Service www.cas.org
Biological Abstracts www.biosis.com

The precise criteria for evaluation will differ according to the information and the subject, but some generally applicable criteria can be outlined. They will generally include factors such as:

- *authority*: who provides the information, and what are their qualifications to do so
- *objectivity*: is the information balanced or biased; does it reflect a particular point of view
- *currency*: how regularly is the information updated; is the age of the information clear
- *accuracy*: how reliable is the information; to what degree of detail; what are the quality control procedures
- *coverage*: what topics are covered; in what depth, and with what degree of balance
- *added value*: does the source provide evaluation, summarization, expert comment, and similar added value, or does it simply provide 'raw' data
- *completeness*: is the coverage intended to be complete, or is it limited in some way, e.g. geographically or by time period
- *format and design*: how appropriate to the type of information being handled

- *access*: what is the convenience and cost of access
- *alternatives*: is this the only source of this information, or is it one of many alternatives?

Issues in, and criteria for, evaluation of sources are reviewed by Bawden (1990) and, specifically for internet sources, by Cooke (1999) and by Alexander & Tate (1999).

References

Alexander J E, Tate M A 1999 Web Wisdom: how to evaluate and create information quality on the web. Lawrence Earlbaum, New York

Bawden D 1999 User-oriented evaluation of information systems and services. Gower, Aldershot

Bawden D 1998 Competitor intelligence in the pharmaceutical industry. Encyclopaedia of Library and Information Sciences 63 (suppl 26): 33–52

Bawden D, Brock A M 1982 Chemical toxicology searching: a collaborative evaluation, comparing information resources and searching techniques. Journal of Information Science 5(1): 3–18

Cooke A 1999 Guide to finding quality information on the internet: selection and evaluation strategies. Library Association Publishing, London

Gretz M, Thomas M 1995 The in-house database – nicety or necessity? Drug Information Journal 29: 161–169

Grogan D 1970 Science and technology; an introduction to the literature. Bingley, London

Krol T F, Coleman J C, Bryant P J 1996 Scientific competitive intelligence in R&D decision making. Drug Information Journal 30: 242–256

Large A, Tedd L A, Hartley R J 1999 Information seeking in the online age: principles and practice. Bowker-Saur, East Grinstead

Malone P M, Mosdell K W, Kier K L, et al 1996 Drug information: a guide for pharmacists. Appleton & Lange Stamford, Connecticut

Morton L T, Godbolt S (eds) 1999 Information sources in the medical sciences. Bowker Saur, London

Mullen 1990 Chemical and physicochemical information In: Pickering W R (ed) Information sources in pharmaceuticals. Bowker Saur, East Grinstead, 11–51

Pickering W R (ed) 1990 Information sources in pharmaceuticals. Bowker Saur, East Grinstead

Robinson L 2000 (a) A strategic approach to research using Internet tools and resources. Aslib Proceedings 52(1): 11–19

Robinson L (b) 2000 Toxicology information: impact of new ICTs on a multidisciplinary science. Paper presented at the 8th International Conference on Medical Librarianship, London

Robinson L, Bawden D 1999 Internet subject gateways. International Journal of Information Management 19(6): 511–522

Robinson L, McIlwaine I, Copestake P, et al 2000 Comparative evaluation of the performance of online databases in answering toxicology queries. International Journal of Information Management, 20(1): 79–99

Sodha R J, van Amelsvoort T 1994 Multi-database searches in biomedicine. Journal of Information Science 20(2): 139–141

Wood M S (ed) 2000 Health care resources on the internet. Haworth Press, New York

Chapter 3

Information technology

Neil Gow, Caroline Holden and Shapour Hariri

Introduction: the effective use of information technology in information work

The pharmaceutical industry and healthcare providers have used computers and information technology for many years now. Typical uses include maintaining patient records and appointment schedules, accessing databases of scientific and medical information, managing an organization's internal information and documents, and office applications such as word-processors and spreadsheets. In the 1970s and 1980s most applications were based on large mainframe computers, using punched cards or 'dumb' terminals to send instructions to the computer. Towards the end of the 1980s and in the 1990s the mainframes and terminals have been largely replaced by desktop personal computers (PCs), connected to a network 'fileserver' for access to shared information. The advances in computing technology mean that the PCs of today are generally more powerful than typical mid-1980s mainframes.

Electronic mail (email) has been a popular form of communication since the 1980s. Initially it was mainly used within large organizations for internal communications at one site. Later, with the availability of packet switching technology, it was used for communication between sites and with other organizations using the same technology. It has proved to be a much faster and more cost-effective method of communication than traditional postal and internal mail services, and is especially useful for communicating with people working in a different time-zone. Now with the development of the internet protocols (TCP/IP and FTP) almost anybody with a computer can use email and send almost any type of document as an attachment for review by another person

The extension of email into teamworking applications has major benefits, especially for large organizations with physically dispersed project teams. Specialized teamworking applications provide the capability for electronic diaries, scheduling of meetings and resources, knowledge-bases and workflow scheduling for projects and documents. These are discussed in the section on communication and teamworking tools.

The internet technologies are having a major impact on how we acquire, manage and distribute information. Commercial databases of information, which used to require special terminal access, are increasingly becoming available on the internet. Within our organizations, internal databases can be accessed via intranets, thus making them available to many more users without the need to install sophisticated software. Internet technologies, through the use of intranets, are also starting to become the backbone of groupware applications. This use of common protocols has particular benefits for communication within and between organizations where different types of computers and networks are employed. The section on internet technologies gives examples of the influence these are having on information management.

Computer databases enable us to store, index and search large volumes of data. One of the best known of the publicly available databases is the Medline biomedical literature database. This is now available via traditional online hosts, on CD-ROM and on the internet. Within our organizations, we use databases to manage scientific, medical and financial data, staff information and document distribution. Development of database technologies has given information professionals an array of sophisticated tools with which to manage and distribute information both internally and externally. These are described in the section on databases, along with some examples of their use.

Document imaging and document management systems are used to store and distribute documents electronically. They enable rapid retrieval of document-based information from large collections, and can even include teamworking and publishing functionality. These are also discussed in the section on databases.

One of the greatest benefits of computer technology is the sheer number-crunching power, the ability to process and analyse large volumes of data in a short time. This is used, for example, in clinical data management. Clinical trials of new pharmaceuticals generate vast amounts of data which must be analysed using sophisticated data handling and statistical applications. Meanwhile, every time a drug is prescribed in a hospital or doctor's surgery, there is the potential to gather data about its benefits and adverse effects through post-marketing surveillance. Systematic gathering and analysis of these data is assisting the new culture of evidence-based medicine, of which the Cochrane Library is one example.

These technologies are making a real difference to the way we work and will continue to do so in the future. In a continuing drive to improve efficiency, pharmaceutical companies have always been early adopters and are often at the forefront of information technology developments. Now also, in the UK National Health Service (NHS), the 1998 government white paper on information strategy for the NHS—*Information for Health* (www.nhsia.nhs.uk/strategy/full/contents.htm)—has highlighted the importance of IT and views it as a central component of other modernization plans.

Communication and teamworking tools

Email, newsgroups and bulletin boards are all examples of communication technologies which make use of modern computer networks. A relatively new term, 'groupware', is used for software that supports multiple users working on related tasks. The term was coined in 1978 by Peter and Trudy Johnson-Lenz, first appeared in print in 1981 (Johnson-Lenz & Johnson-Lenz 1981) and was described as 'Intentional group processes plus software to support them'. Often used for particular packages, notably Lotus Notes and Microsoft Exchange, the term can also be applied to other software applications that facilitate shared work on documents and information.

The development of groupware has paralleled the increasing use within organizations of 'virtual teams'. These are flexible teams which can be assembled and disbanded quickly yet which can solve problems efficiently and effectively. These teams can be categorized into 'co-located', where users are physically together and work face-to-face, and 'distance' or 'dispersed' where they are in different locations, and may even be in different countries. In order for these virtual teams to work effectively they need to have easy and flexible access to other team members and information, and to be able to hold meetings. The groupware tools are designed for distributed group-member use. They can be easily accessed by the team members at any time and from any place, avoiding the problems of geographical separation and time-zone differences, and help to speed up the decision-making processes.

Groupware applications and technologies

Groupware technologies may be classified by whether they support 'real-time' or 'asynchronous' groups, as demonstrated in Table 3.1.

The use of effective groupware applications offers benefits such as improved and faster communications, reduced travel costs and time and improved group problem-solving.

Some of the technologies and applications used for communication and teamworking are now considered in more detail.

Table 3.1 *Uses of groupware applications*

Type of Group	Real-time (synchronous) groups	Asynchronous groups
Examples of group activities	Marketing staff using a shared drawing surface to edit or annotate an advertisement	Passing a manuscript from one team member to another for review and comment
	Virtual meeting	Updating a centralized workplan
Examples of applications	Real-time data conferencing Videoconferencing	Workflow applications Project team folders

Email

Electronic mail, or email, is the transmission of text-based messages between networked computers. It is the most widely used communication application (after the telephone). Although the basic function is to pass messages between two users, most programs allow additional features such as forwarding and filing messages, creation of mailing groups and inclusion of files such as word processing documents, programs, audio and video, and graphics, as attachments to the message. Some systems also allow automatic sorting and processing, for example 'out of the office' messages, automatic routing and structured communication.

Email addresses have two basic components, a user name and the user's location or 'domain' name, e.g. membership@aiopi.org.uk. Every location (mail-server) has a unique domain name. Sometimes this leads to email addresses becoming quite long but many organizations now have aliasing systems in place so that the domain name part of the email address can be abbreviated.

Newsgroups and mailing lists

These are similar to email systems but are intended for messages to large groups of users. Both use special software which allows automation of some of the email functions. Both are widely used amongst patient groups and within specialized medical sites on the worldwide web.

Mailing lists deliver messages via email, as soon as they become available. A message sent to a list is copied and then forwarded by email to every subscriber. Subscribers can contribute actively by posting messages themselves or they can just read those that others post when they arrive by email. One disadvantage of these systems is that subscribers will continue to receive email messages automatically unless they make a request to be removed from the list.

Newsgroups show messages to a user on demand. An example is USENET, an electronic bulletin board of over 5000 different topic-based news or discussion groups. Special newsreader software allows a user to browse articles on the system and to enter or 'post' an article which can be read by other participants. Most newsreaders allow 'threading' where articles can be read by topic (thread) rather than just in the order in which they are posted. Messages appearing in newsgroups are entered directly by users, and do not undergo any form of checking, although many newsgroups have a 'moderator' who can remove inappropriate messages. The advantage of newsgroups over mailing lists is that users select the messages they want to read rather than having them swamping their mailboxes.

Electronic diaries and scheduling tools

Specialist software, for example Lotus Notes, Microsoft Outlook, Corel Groupwise and Schedule Plus, are available to help in the planning and scheduling of group activities, tracking progress and coordinating the activities of individual members. Typical features allow detection of scheduling conflicts and the identification of available meeting times for all essential participants. They may also be used to schedule resources such as meeting rooms and cars. These systems can save a great deal of time, but to function effectively they require the commitment of all group members. If some users are not convinced that the time it takes to keep their calendars up to date is justified by the benefits to the group then the system will break down.

These software packages also form the basis of computer conferencing systems. Team members can post messages to their 'team folder' on the email/diary server , check to see what has changed since they last logged in and make comments if required. The system can also be used for processing drafts of documents.

Workflow applications

Workflow applications allow documents to be routed through organizations via a formal process, e.g. expense forms or documents requiring review. They may provide features such as routing, development of forms and support for differing roles and privileges. They can provide asynchronous support where the software shows authorship of documents and allows users to track changes and make annotations to the document. In some cases authors will be given additional tools which help plan and coordinate the authoring process, such as being able to link to other documents.

Basic workflow can be implemented in the familiar email/scheduling applications such as Lotus Notes and Microsoft Outlook. More sophisticated workflow may include parallel routing (documents being reviewed by more than one person simultaneously), version control and notification of tasks not completed by the required date. These are found in more sophisticated document management systems such as Documentum and Opentext Livelink, discussed later in this chapter.

Knowledgebases

Knowledgebases are designed to allow information to be shared throughout organizations and support collaboration over local and wide area networks (LANs and WANs). They provide a centralized archive and conferencing facilities which enable users to add comments (responses) to previous entries, thus promoting online discussions and knowledge sharing. Multi-layered security can be applied so that different classes of users can be allowed access to separate parts of the database. One of the best known is Lotus Notes, which also allows users to attach documents such as copies of standard letters or spreadsheets of data to their entries.

Some conventional databases used for storing information are sometimes referred to as knowledgebases, as are technical support or 'frequently asked questions' (FAQ) pages on some websites. Neither of these are true knowledgebases as they lack the facility for sharing further knowledge on a subject through reader responses and discussion threads..

Synchronous or 'real-time' groupware

Desktop and real-time data conferencing are shared workspace facilities which enable multiple users to see and work with documents simultaneously. They include electronic whiteboards and shared screen facilities which enable part of an individual's screen to be reproduced on one or more remote screens. Collaborative writing tools with synchronous support enable users to see each other's changes as they are made.

In computer-supported data conferencing each member of the team has a networked computer. Team members are able to work privately or to display their work for others to see during the meeting. This has led to custom-designed meeting rooms, called teamrooms, containing groupware applications which support a range of meeting requirements such as decision support systems, brainstorming and presentation software. These applications are often designed to encourage equal participation by providing anonymity or enforcing turn-taking.

Adding audio and video communications to the data conferencing environment can improve productivity further. Audio increases the effectiveness of text-based communication because added information is provided through intonation and accent, and this can help in interpretation. Tools combining telephone and shared computer facilities can improve the effectiveness of non face-to-face meetings. They enable meetings to be carried out while members remain in their own offices. Information from any team member can be presented on a screen and then discussed by all members of the group.

Video can be used to support task-related working when group members are dispersed. The use of images in addition to audio facilitates spontaneous interaction and informal communication between team members, enabling them to 'get to know' each other. These interactions are important to the normal dynamics of team working and are not possible with other groupware applications. For real-time applications special software and hardware are needed to avoid transmission bandwidth problems which result in break-up of the image or jerky images. The systems that exist are expensive because of the technology required to handle the large volumes of data which need to be transmitted. For this reason videoconferencing is usually carried out in special rooms set aside for this purpose, or it may be one of the facilities available in a teamroom (see above).

Table 3.2 demonstrates how groupware can improve productivity.

Intranet groupware

As the internet and intranets become more commonplace it is being suggested that 'traditional' groupware may become obsolete. Vendors of traditional groupware are increasingly making their products web-friendly so that they can take advantage of the benefits that this technology offers. Examples are the email and electronic diary systems provided by Microsoft and Netscape, both of which are tightly integrated with their respective web browser software and are extending their capabilities to add teamworking facilities such as team folders. A further development is the release of a version of Lotus Notes (the knowledgebase example mentioned above) with a fully web-functional interface. Called Lotus Notes Domino, this retains the functionality of previous versions while providing a much more standard and intuitive interface for users.

Table 3.2 *Organizing a project team meeting – before and after groupware*

Before	After
Telephone each team member for available dates. Find suitable date and telephone each again to confirm meeting date. Time taken, 2 hours.	Run a search on the electronic diary system to find a time when everyone is available and schedule meeting electronically. Time taken, 15 minutes.
Photocopy and post out meeting agenda and minutes of previous meeting to all team members. Time taken, 30 minutes.	Attach meeting agenda and minutes documents to the meeting appointment. Time taken, 5 minutes.
Telephone each team member to seek an opinion on one issue you know will be thorny. Repeat process to make each member aware of the views of others. Time taken, 2 hours.	Remind team members by email to check the discussion database and provide responses to the thorny issue that has been raised there. Time taken, 5 minutes.
Telephone team members to check if they have completed outstanding actions. Time taken, 30 minutes.	Check project discussion database for uncompleted actions. Remind appropriate team members by email. Time taken, 5 minutes.
Gather together copies of previous minutes, documents etc. Update project file. Time taken, 1 hour.	All project documents are in the project discussion database. Time taken, nil.
Spend your time making telephone calls and copying pieces of paper.	Spend your time actually managing and progressing the project.

Internet, intranets and extranets

The internet—definition and history

The internet is a worldwide system of computer networks. It interconnects a very large number of compatible publicly accessible networks through high-speed links on a global scale. It allows a user to communicate privately and publicly, send and retrieve information and find and view information. It has two main components, email and the worldwide web (WWW or 'the web'). In the space of a very few years it has altered the way people work and it has revolutionized the way that businesses communicate with the outside world and share information internally.

The internet grew out of an experimental network, called the ARPANET, built for the US government in 1969 and initially linking four US academic centres. This was based on a 'packet-switch' network, where data is broken into small pieces or 'packets' which can be forwarded by other computers ('servers') on the network in any order and which are labelled in such a way that they can be reassembled once they reach their destination. Packet-switching allows users to send information across networks efficiently and simultaneously and, one of the main requirements for ARPANET, it means that if one or more of the connecting servers are unavailable data can be re-routed and the network will continue to function. During the 1970s the ARPANET carried much of the day-to-day US Department of Defense network traffic, and the TCP/IP network protocol used today was developed. In 1983 the military sites were split off from ARPANET and it became a purely civilian network. The National Science Foundation (NSF) then took up the baton and created the NSFNET, based on ARPANET protocols, to provide a national backbone service free to any US research or educational institution.

Today the internet is a public facility accessible to hundreds of millions of people worldwide. Physically it uses a part of the resources of the currently existing telecommunications networks, using a network protocol called TCP/IP (Transmission Control Protocol / Internet Protocol). Another protocol, called FTP (File Transfer Protocol), is used for transferring files from one computer to another over the internet. It can be used to download files, including software, product upgrades and information. In order to connect to a remote computer it used to be necessary to know the exact address, and have a user ID and password. Now many computers have been made publicly accessible by the use of 'anonymous FTP access', which allows any user to enter and then download files. In many cases it is no longer necessary to know the address of the FTP server, as it can be accessed via a hyperlink from a web page.

Email and newsgroups

For many people the use of email is now as routine as the written postal service, and has become the preferred method for sending short written transactions. A fuller discussion of email and newsgroups is included under the 'Communication and teamworking tools' heading in this chapter. There have been a number of email systems over the years, but it is the internet technologies and in particular the adoption of the standard TCP/IP network protocol and SMTP mail protocol which has been responsible for the recent rapid growth in use of email and newsgroups. Now everyone is talking the same language. The internet has enabled the extension of email and teamworking applications to an external environment

The worldwide web

After email, the most widely used part of the internet is the worldwide web. This provides a uniform user-friendly interface to the internet. Information is displayed as pages of multimedia objects that can include text, graphics, audio and video. The pages are linked together with hypertext pointers which allow data stored in computers anywhere on the internet (i.e. anywhere in the world) to be viewed from a user's computer. As the information can be located anywhere the user is exploring a 'web' of information rather than a tree-like hierarchical structure.

The term worldwide web was first used in 1990 by Tim Berners-Lee at CERN, and the first WWW 'browser' (software which allows web pages to be viewed) was installed at CERN in 1991 (World Wide Web consortium 1995). The web started its phenomenal growth in late 1993 when the first commercial browser called Mosaic was released. The components of the web technologies are listed in Table 3.3.

The use of the internet by the pharmaceutical industry

The healthcare industry accounts for one of the largest commercial sectors on the web. Both professionals and patients already make extensive use of this medium and there are very many sites and discussion groups on medicine-related topics.

The first pharmaceutical company sites were set up to provide information to investors and contained financial information, annual reports and press releases, along with advertisements for employment. This type of information is often still given prominence over other information present on an industry site. This may be because the pharmaceutical industry was quick to recognize that the financial sector was using the internet to research investment opportunities and look at market data. In addition, the internet offers a convenient and economical way of distributing annual reports and quarterly figures on a global scale.

One reason for the initial lack of product-related information in pharmaceutical company sites is uncertainty about what information can be made available to the general public. Companies have been hesitant about putting information on prescription products onto the web in case they are regarded as advertising such products to the general public. Some have

Table 3.3 *Components of the worldwide web*

Component	Definition
Hypertext	The basis of the web. Enables any sort of digital data to be distributed inside a document. Provides the mechanism for links to other documents.
Hypertext transfer protocol (HTTP)	This is the protocol used to transfer hypertext information on the web.
Hypertext markup language (HTML)	The language of the web. Defines the appearance of the document by tagging certain areas so that a browser will display them in a certain way. Also defines hyperlink and graphic image properties. HTML editors are available to simplify the writing of HTML. A more structured version called XML (extensible markup language) is now starting to appear.
Uniform resource locator (URL)	The standard form of address used in hypertext links. They are used to ensure every web page has a unique name and also to interact with other web services such as file transfer protocol (FTP) and email. Most URLs contain 3 pieces of information, the protocol to be used, the internet address or host name of the server and the file path to follow to access the required file.
Internet service provider (ISP)	Organization which has suitable servers and IP (internet protocol) addresses to host web sites. There are many commercial ISPs to choose from. Large companies and academic institutions host their own sites rather than use a commercial ISP.
Web browser	Software used to retrieve and display web documents. The two most commonly used are Netscape Navigator and Microsoft's Internet Explorer.

tackled this issue by creating password-protected sections of their site containing information designed for a specific user group such as medical practitioners. Others have sponsored general medical sites or sites devoted to a specific disease area, managed by a patient group. Some of the successful ones include Roche's HIV website (http://www.roche-hiv.com), Novartis's Café Herpé (http://www.cafeherpe.com), and Eli Lilly's Managing your Diabetes (http://diabetes.lilly.com). Some medical information departments now have their own password protected sites for medics and pharmacists which offer standard medical information services aiming to cut down the number of enquiries received by telephone. These sites contain frequently asked questions about the companies' products and offer email links for additional queries. They also contain product information, including updates, and are therefore more current than the printed versions.

Pharmaceutical companies, like others, are also using the internet as a source of information. Both the research communities and medical information departments can benefit from the wealth of information on the WWW. There are now so many sites dedicated to health and medicine that products such as Caredata's Citeline are being developed to help search and navigate through these. Some of the types of information resources available on the internet are summarized in Table 3.4.

Table 3.4 *Types of information resource on the internet*

Type of site	Types of information available	Examples
Publishers/Journal sites	Contents pages. Full text articles (usually restricted to subscribers only). Guide for authors.	ScienceDirect, http://www.sciencedirect.com Highwire Press, http://highwire.stanford.edu
Literature/Medical databases	Medline free via Pubmed and several other locations. Other databases available via subscription.	Pubmed, http://www.ncbi.nlm.nih.gov/ PubMed Embase.com, http://embase.com/about
Third-party access to journal articles	Database of articles with links to publishers' sites for subscribers and pay-per-view facility for non-subscribers.	Ingenta, http://www.ingenta.com
Semi-official bodies and charities	Epidemiology information. Reviews of treatments, clinical trials and ongoing research.	Imperial Cancer Research Fund, http://www.icnet.uk
Regulatory authorities	Regulations and guidelines can be downloaded as documents. Searching facility provided.	Food and Drug Administration, http://www.fda.gov European Medicines Evaluation Agency, http://www.emea.eu.int
Patent authorities	Search for patents and download copies of complete patent documents.	US Patent and Trademarks Office, http://www.uspto.gov/patft European Patent Office, http://www.european-patent-office.org
Hub sites (web communities)	Subject sites offering a range of facilities and links for members	BioMedNet, http://www.biomednet.com/map PharmWeb, http://www.pharmweb.net

The use of the internet by the National Health Service in the UK

The UK National Health Service (NHS) has been slower to adopt the internet, and hospitals have just recently started to offer internet access to their employees. However, the internet is used extensively by NHS information services to search for information using some of the information sources mentioned above. Publishing of information on the internet by NHS organizations is also gathering pace and new health-related websites are launched every day. Email is becoming a standard method of communication and will be a considerable improvement for individuals scattered throughout sites across the UK. An example of this is the UK DI mailing list, which is a closed, moderated mailing list used by drug information (DI) pharmacists in the UK. DI pharmacists use this mailing list to communicate with other colleagues and share information and experiences.

Limitations of the internet

The internet offers many benefits to users within the healthcare industry, as outlined above, but it has some limitations.

One technical issue is the speed and reliability of connections. The internet is only as strong as the weakest link in the chain and with the ever increasing numbers of users slow access times could become even more of a problem. Although the technologies involved are being improved to take account of this (high-bandwidth transmission systems and data compression amongst them) they may well struggle to keep pace with the growth in internet use.

Another serious consideration is that of security and privacy. The main backbone of the internet uses public data networks, and there is a real potential for interception of private information. Company confidential, financial and personal information are all examples of information which must be protected from possible interception. There are now methods for increasing the security of data transmitted over the internet and these are becoming increasingly used. These include data encryption, the use of a secure sockets layer (SSL) and the use of private leased lines for data transmission.

One key issue regarding its content is the varied quality of information available. Although the internet contains much information that is up to date and valuable, it also contains information that is out of date and inaccurate. The user must decide how much faith to place in the source of any data, but some will be less able to make this judgement and could be misled. Several attempts have been made at publishing criteria for evaluating health-related web sites (Kim et al 1999).

In countries such as the UK widespread use of the internet can lead to conflict between patients and their health providers. Patients who use the internet to locate information on particular treatments or procedures may start to demand specific treatment from their health service, regardless of cost or suitability. This has prompted the UK Prescription Medicines Code of Practice Authority to issue guidance explaining where companies need to be cautious when using the internet. Even if pharmaceutical companies avoid openly promoting their products, disease support groups may do it for them, as was the case with Viagra in 1999. There is also potential for confusion when a product is marketed with different indications in different countries, as the information retrieved by an internet user is global.

Future developments of the internet

It seems clear that in the future even more pharmaceutical information will become available to the general public over the internet. Healthcare generally is moving towards a more patient-orientated strategy and the internet is an ideal tool for disseminating the information that patients require to make informed decisions. In addition, more and more healthcare professionals are using the internet on a routine basis as a source of general background information on a product.

as the clinical data must remain blinded (i.e. it is not known which patients received the trial drug and which received placebo or a comparative drug) until the study is complete.

Data analysis is performed using a separate program. Almost universally a program called SAS (http://www.sas.com) is used. This is the industry standard for the pharmaceutical industry and is also used by the US Food and Drug Administration. Data are exported from the database, using tools provided or developed in-house, to files that SAS can read. SAS will then perform a statistical analysis and produce reports.

A typical process for gathering and processing data is as follows. The clinician completes a case report form (CRF), which includes the protocol and study number, patient ID and outcome of the drug administration. The clinical research associate collects the CRFs during a visit to the clinical centre and takes them to the company site. Some companies will scan the CRFs into a database of digitized documents at this stage, as they constitute important raw data; others may microfilm them. A team of data entry personnel will enter the data from the forms into the database, usually working overnight and at weekends. When a study reaches its endpoint the company statisticians (biometricians) will run reports from the database to produce data files for analysis by SAS. Meanwhile the SAS programmers will have been writing programs that analyse the data in the most appropriate way for the clinical endpoint under investigation, and to produce clear and meaningful reports.

The end result of all this activity is a study report. The Regulatory Affairs department will compile this into a dossier along with other study reports and any required preclinical and manufacturing data, for submission to the regulatory authorities. This is part of the document management process and is another area where IT plays a pivotal role with tools such as Documentum and CoreDossier.

Use of information technology within the UK NHS

The United Kingdom National Health Service (NHS) makes use of information technology in a number of ways. Many of these have been mentioned in the text above but a summary is provided here for completeness.

Information strategy for the NHS

Modernizing the NHS is a central theme to the current UK government's programme. The government's information strategy for the NHS was set out in the September 1998 white paper, *Information for Health* (www.nhsia.nhs.uk/strategy/full/contents.htm). This document highlights the importance of information technology in the future of the NHS and views it as a central component of other NHS modernizing plans.

Information for Health is a seven-year strategy that sets out an ambitious programme of IT developments for the NHS. It is however backed by the pledge of £1bn of new money over the next seven years and part of the NHS £5bn modernization fund. The main components are listed below.

Electronic health record (EHR)

EHR is the concept of creating a lifelong electronic record of a patient's health and his or her interactions with the NHS. Since the majority of patient contact is in primary care it is proposed that the majority of the information contained within the EHR will be from primary care with summary information from secondary care sources. Such an electronic record will allow NHS staff instant access to patient records, 24 hours a day. Anonymized subsets of the data will be used for research and management.

Electronic patient records (EPR)

It is acknowledged that only a small number of acute NHS Trusts have implemented EPR to various degrees of sophistication and this is far from ideal. The EPR will record information about the treatment and care that individual patients receive in hospital. The strategy proposes that over seven years all NHS trusts must implement specified minimum level EPR systems. It is also envisaged that summaries from the EPRs will be added to the Electronic Health Record (EHR) of patients.

NHSnet

NHSnet is a secure computer network for the NHS and is based on internet technology. As mentioned earlier in the chapter, NHSnet is a wide area network (WAN) linking the local area networks in hospitals and other NHS organizations. It is intended to become an 'information superhighway' for NHS messages and information. However the government also acknowledges the potential of the internet and a one-way link to the internet will be provided through NHSnet. At present NHSnet is poor in content, access and bandwidth but the NHS is assured that improvement will take place over the next few years.

National electronic library for health (NeLH)

The NeLH (http://www.nelh.nhs.uk) intends to take advantage of the rapid expansion of electronic media to help healthcare professionals in accessing reference material. It aims to be the single most comprehensive source of medical reference material in the UK and to make resources and information accessible at the 'bedside' or 'desktop'.

Information services for patients and the public

The present NHS Direct is a 24–hour national helpline and is an increasingly important vehicle for providing health information to members of the public. It is envisaged that new technology such as internet technology will be used to allow NHS Direct to act as a convenient home-based gateway to the NHS.

Telemedicine and telecare

Telemedicine is a healthcare-related activity involving a professional and a patient (or one professional and another) who are separated in space, facilitated by the use of information technology. Telecare is similar but is delivered in the patient's home. Telemedicine can be used by general practitioners to obtain rapid second opinions from disease specialists. A telemedicine program called Dermaclinic has been piloted and initial reports (D'Souza et al 1999) indicate that the number of referrals to outpatients and treatment waiting times are both reduced.

These technologies may also be used to reduce unnecessary travel and delays for patients by providing direct online access to NHS services and expertise.

The UK drug information network (see Chapter 8) will have an active and necessary role to play in all the above components. The maintenance of drug knowledgebases in EPR programs and decision support systems should be the responsibility of drug information pharmacists. The drug information component of the NeLH is an ideal area for involvement of drug information pharmacists.

Use of IT in the UK drug information (UKDI) network

As with medical information departments within the pharmaceutical industry, the drug information centres rely heavily on a wide range of IT resources for information retrieval and analysis. Regional drug information centres have access to a wide variety of biomedical databases, reference sources and the internet. Each regional and local drug information centre is required to comply with a minimum IT specification as described in the UK drug information manual (Judd 1997).

The United Kingdom Drug Information Pharmacists Group (UKDIPG), which leads and coordinates drug information practice in the UK, in 1999 published a five-year strategy for drug information. In view of future government plans for the NHS and its IT policies, the strategy predicts a move away from passive enquiry answering towards active knowledge generation. DI pharmacists will be expected to be key in the development and maintenance of drug knowledgebases which will be at the heart of modern decision support and electronic prescribing systems. Drug information centres will also be responsible for the delivery of accurate and up-to-date drug information at the point of prescribing. These goals can only be achieved if information management technology is utilized effectively.

An important initiative by United Kingdom Drug Information Pharmacists Group (UKDIPG) has been the development of Pharm-Line®, a bibliographical database focused on the clinical use of drugs and pharmacy practice. Over 100 pharmacy and biomedical journals are scanned every month and articles are selected and abstracted and keywords are assigned according to agreed criteria. The database is distributed on CD-ROM and NHSnet and utilises a powerful Boolean search engine. The database software in Pharm-Line® is also being used to share bulletins, drug evaluations and other appropriate reports produced by regional DI centres. It is envisaged that this database can grow to form a national frequently asked questions (FAQ) database with model answers to common DI enquiries.

Conclusion

Considering all the topics in this chapter, it is clear that there is a vast array of IT tools available to today's information managers, which when used effectively enable us to improve productivity and the distribution of information. It is also clear that this is a rapidly moving field, and if anything the pace of technology change is faster today that it has ever been, so the future looks very exciting indeed.

It must be emphasized though, that IT only provides the tools to enable us to develop faster and better access to information. For evidence that these tools require skilled professionals for their effective use, just look at the internet. More than half the websites you will ever visit are poor in content, poor in design and difficult to navigate. However good the technology gets, the skills of the information professional will always be required to ensure that the appropriate information is presented to users in a properly structured environment that facilitates easy selection.

References

Date C J 1994 An Introduction to database systems 6th edn. Addison-Wesley, Reading, Massachussetts

D'Souza M, Shah D, Misch K, et al 1999 Dermatology opinions via intranet could reduce waiting times. British Medical Journal 318: 737

Johnson-Lenz P, Johnson-Lenz T 1981 Consider the groupware: design and group process impacts on communication in the electronic medium. In: Hiltz S, Kerr E Studies of computer-mediated communications systems: a synthesis of the findings research report number 16 Computerized Conferencing and Communications Center. New Jersey Institute of Technology, Newark, New Jersey

Judd A (ed) 1997 UK Drug Information Manual, 4th edn. UK Drug Information Pharmacists Group, Leeds (available from: Drugs and Poisons Information Service, The General Infirmary, Great George Street, Leeds LS1 3EX, UK)

Kim P, Eng T R, Deering M J, et al 1999 Published criteria for evaluating web related sites: review. British Medical Journal 318: 647–649

Shipman A (ed) 1996 Code of practice for legal admissibility of information stored on electronic data management systems. British Standards Institution DISC PD0008

World Wide Web consortium. A little history of the world wide web. http://www.w3c.rl.ac.uk/talks/lectures/14Resources/01/01MiniHistory.htm; 1995.

Further Reading

Lloyd P. Groupware in the 21st Century: Computer Supported Cooperative Working Toward the Millennium. London: Adamantine Press; 1994.

London & South East drug information web site: http://www.druginfozone.org

Montlick T What is Object-Oriented Software: http://www.soft-design.com/softinfo/objects.html, accessed 2nd November 1999.

NHS information authority web site: http://www.doh.gov.uk/nhsexipu/index.htm

United Kingdom Drug Information Pharmacist Group web site: http://www.ukdipg.org.uk

Webopedia dictionary of IT Terms: http://webopedia.internet.com/

Chapter 4

Information and knowledge management

David Bawden and Elizabeth Orna

Introduction

The purpose of this chapter is to introduce some of the main concepts and issues in the management of information and knowledge, and to show their importance in a pharmaceutical setting.

Pharmaceuticals is an area which has long been known as 'information intensive', with a diverse range of external and internal sources requiring effective management (see, for example, Brown 1983, Haygarth-Jackson 1977, 1987). Some of the particular factors contributing to this are:

- the multidisciplinary nature of pharmaceutical research and development, and of the subsequent marketing and use of medicines
- the diverse and expanding basic science knowledge base
- an increasingly globalized and competitive situation
- increasing regulation, and increased consumer awareness.

Overviews of information management in pharmaceutical settings are given by Abbott (1998), and by Henderson (1994), who argues that pharmaceutical companies have a unique managerial competence of fostering a high level of specialized knowledge within the organization while preventing that information base from fixing the company in the past. Dieckmann & Whittall (1998) and Hamilton (1997) give accounts of information management in individual companies.

The chapter is divided into eight sections, following this introduction. The first three sections deal with basic disciplines within the information and knowledge management framework: information resource management; knowledge management; and knowledge organization. The next three sections deal with three significant processes: information mapping and auditing; developing information policies and strategies; and valuing information. The final two sections deal with issues of current importance: information overload and information literacy.

Information and knowledge

It is difficult, and unnecessary for the purposes of this chapter, to make a sharp distinction between the two concepts of information and knowledge. It is better to consider a spectrum of forms of information, from data, through information with varying degrees of structure, to knowledge, and perhaps wisdom. This is conventionally drawn as a pyramid, to suggest that knowledge is somehow a higher form, and lesser in volume, but this may sometimes be misleading.

Moving through this spectrum, from information to knowledge, involves various structuring processes, which can be described in general as 'value-adding'—evaluation, comparison, compilation, classification, and so on. Knowledge can then be seen as that form of information characterized by compression, abstraction, categorization, and contexualization, and which is thereby endowed with meaning and significance, and transformative power.

Various approaches to quantifying the degree of added value, and hence the extent of transformation of information into knowledge, have been proposed, though none has been generally accepted. Some relate to the effort or cost of the transformation. Others, stemming from studies in the theory of computation, describe the 'logical depth' of the information, i.e. the number of steps necessary to recreate the original information. (Thus a scientific law of nature, a prime example of abstract knowledge, would have a large logical depth, since it would take a considerable number of steps to create from this the data from a measuring instrument.)

An alternative view of the information / knowledge dichotomy is to think of knowledge as being the form of information possessed by an individual, since only a thinking individual can recognize meaning and significance. Information is then the means by which knowledge is transferred between individuals, while knowledge management is primarily a matter of dealing with the personal knowledge, and hence it is a matter of culture as much as, or more than, of systems and technologies.

One consequence of this is that it is not feasible to make a sharp distinction between information management and associated disciplines; the link with knowledge management is discussed below, and that with records management by Goodman (1994).

Foundations for information management

In order to think about the three interlinked areas of information auditing, information policy and information value, we need a strategic understanding of the organization's business and of the implications for what it needs to know and how it should use information and knowledge. The answers to three key questions provide a foundation:

- what do the people who work for this organization need to know in order to act to achieve its objectives?
- what information resources do they need to maintain their knowledge?
- in using information and applying knowledge, how do they need to interact with information, with one another and with the organization's 'outside world' ?

Pharmaceutical exemplification

A pharmaceutical example, based on real-life case studies carried out by one of the chapter authors, will be used throughout this chapter to give context to the general points made.

Three key objectives of a large research-based pharmaceutical firm are:

- to identify new compounds for exploratory research
- through the research and development programme, to determine which compounds have appropriate safety and efficacy
- to bring these compounds to registration.

To meet these objectives, the company has a number of knowledge and know-how requirements.

General areas of knowledge required:

- medical research
- health service
- markets (actual and potential)
- pharmaceutical industry
- competitors and their products
- social and economic environment
- company's own past and current research
- company's critical success factors for evaluating exploratory research proposals
- developments in research methods and technologies
- regulatory requirements, institutions, relevant legislation
- customers
- suppliers
- knowledge of sources and skills in searching them
- relevant developments in higher education.

Information resources to maintain required knowledge:

- relevant databases
- periodicals
- abstracting services
- statistical series
- market reports
- competitor intelligence service
- government publications
- database of company's own research projects, accessible on company intranet
- Human Resources database with answers to questions such as: who knows about ...? who has skills in ...? who has training in ...?
- contacts database
- customer database
- conference reports
- company's own information products, internal and external
- supporting systems/IT infrastructure, including intranet and WWW access.

Necessary information flows and interactions for making use of knowledge and information:

In-house

- researchers
- information/knowledge specialists
- systems/IT
- HR
- legal
- sales
- marketing
- senior management.

External

- customers
- suppliers
- professional and trade bodies

- researchers in other companies
- regulatory institutions.

This is where the process gets interesting, and the answers become illuminating but lengthy. Readers in the pharmaceutical industry may like to add to/amend the above list, and then work out the information interactions needed, together with the support they require from the organizational structure and from information systems/IT!

Information resource management

It is now customary, in information management circles, to regard information as a resource. Hence the term 'information resource management'. Information is sometimes described more specifically as the 'fourth resource', by analogy with the other three main kinds of resource, which may be possessed by an organization: material, human, and financial.

In as much as this description is taken as being simply a recognition that information is valuable, and should be managed carefully, this can only be good. When the analogy is pressed too hard, however, difficulties appear. Some commentators argue that information should not be regarded as a resource at all, but something more like a public good. If information is indeed a resource, it is rather different in kind from others, being intangible and transformative in character. Most crucially, the value (as distinct from the cost) of information, being entirely dependent on context and use, may be inherently unpredictable. The divergences of the nature of the information resource from others become more pronounced as we move from data towards knowledge.

If we want to treat information as a resource like any other, we must assume that information possesses several clear and definite qualities. Typical is the list given by Eaton & Bawden (1991):

- information is acquired at a definite measurable cost
- information possesses a definite value, which may be quantified and treated as an accountable asset
- information can be consumed, and its consumption can be quantified
- cost-accounting techniques can be applied to help control the costs of information
- information has identifiable and measurable characteristics
- information has a clear life-cycle: definition of requirements, collection, transmission, processing, storage, dissemination, use, disposal
- information may be processed and refined, so that raw materials (e.g. databases) are converted into finished products (e.g. published directories)
- substitutes for any specific items or collection of information are available, and may be quantified as more or less expensive
- choices are available to management in making trade-offs between different grades, types and prices for information.

While some of these assumptions are uncontroversial, taken as a whole this list is unrealistic, except perhaps for certain limited types of information, such as office records.

Information possesses certain unique, even paradoxical, qualities. Examples of these qualities (Eaton & Bawden 1991) are:

- although information is instantiated in physical objects, information itself is intangible, a collection of 'abstract objects'
- information is expandable, increasing with use
- information is compressible, able to be summarized, integrated, etc.
- information can substitute for any other resource in many circumstances
- information is transportable virtually instantaneously

- information is diffusive, tending to leak from the straitjacket of security and control, and the more it leaks the more there is, as new information is created through integration and 'cross-fertilization
- information is sharable, not exchangeable, it can be given away and retained at the same time.

In particular, the value of information, unlike that of other resources, cannot be quantified in any straightforward way, except in special cases. Most approaches to 'information accounting' rely on assessing the cost of acquiring or replacing the information. Information has no intrinsic value, its worth being entirely subjective, depending upon its context and intended use by particular persons on particular occasions. The value of information (see p. 52) cannot therefore be determined in advance, nor does its use, and therefore value, change with time in any regular or predictable manner. Although some types of information, typically 'simple' records, have a well-defined life cycle, most information and knowledge does not.

Nor is the consumption of information similar to that of other resources, since it is not lost when given to others. Nor does it diminish when consumed; on the contrary, wide use of information generally leads to an overall increase in its amount, as users compare and consolidate, leading to the creation of new information. The same item of information may be used by, and have a different value to, an arbitrary large number of users. Unlike other resources, information is self-multiplicative; its exchange does not imply either loss or simple redistribution.

Finally, information and knowledge cannot realistically be regarded as a static resource, to be accumulated and stored. It has a formative, self-organizing character, with the capability to change the organization or society within which it exists. (The word itself, after all, comes from the Latin 'informare', to give form to.)

These considerations suggest that the management of the information resource needs rather different treatment from others, particularly in the assignment of a financial value. This viewpoint does not always make information managers popular with their organizations, but ignoring it does not do justice to the nature of this particular resource.

Since we view knowledge as a particular kind of information, with particular properties, it follows that knowledge management will be a subset of the larger field of information management. It also follows that we do not accept the view that knowledge is a kind of mystical fluid, not amenable to any kind of management.

Information with lower levels of structure, including raw data—which is to say the great majority of information—is generally managed by systems. These systems may be technical (computer hardware and software, card catalogues, etc.) or administrative (procedures, standards, codes of practice, retrieval languages etc.)

Knowledge is too abstract and contextualized to be managed in this way (see p. 50). It can only be managed by policies; generalized principles incorporating the values and vision of an organization or society. There is, therefore, a close link between information policy formulation and the emerging discipline of knowledge management.

Furthermore, it is clear that knowledge management is intrinsically more complex than most of information management. Information and knowledge can be described at four levels: empiric, concerned with the mechanisms of transmission; syntactic, concerned with the languages and codes used; semantic, concerned with meaning; and pragmatic, concerned with significance and application. Though this may seem somewhat abstruse, it is of very practical usefulness in understanding many issues in information management; not least the failings of many IT systems, when solutions at the technical (empiric/syntactic) level were presented for problems involving user-oriented (semantic/pragmatic) issues of meaning and use of information.

Information and IT management may operate at any of these four levels, but typically involve one or two of the lower levels; the levels at which a systems approach is appropriate. Knowledge management and, associated with it, information policy formulation, must necessarily involve the pragmatic, i.e. the highest, level, since this is the level of meaning, which we have noted as a crucial attribute of knowledge. However, a full understanding of this level may require analysis of any of the other levels; hence an intrinsic, and unavoidable complexity.

Knowledge management

Knowledge is classification. (John Dewey)

Knowledge management (hereafter KM) is an over-used term, with many slightly varied definitions. During the late 1990s it was one of the most discussed issues in management, associated with such ideas as the learning organization, the knowledge-based company, and the leverage of intellectual assets.

For our purposes, it can best be regarded as a variant on, and extension of, information management. Its major feature is that it deals with a kind of 'soft', 'tacit' or 'implicit' information—'knowing how', 'knowing who' and 'knowing why'—often ignored by conventional information systems, which concentrate on hard facts and figures. This means that KM is very much concerned with informal, personal, and subjective, knowledge.

Quite what is involved in KM is a matter for debate. Initially, there was strong emphasis on technology as a means towards promoting the sharing of knowledge, using tools such as intranet, groupware, and indexes of individual expertise. It is now generally agreed that cultural aspects are equally, if not more, important. In this view, the most important aspect is to promote, and facilitate, a willingness to share knowledge; this may require attention to issues as diverse as reward systems, and the design of coffee rooms. There is still, however, a reluctance to give due weight to knowledge content and organization.

It is best to regard KM as comprising three linked aspects:

- *Technical*: the means by which knowledge may be stored, retrieved and communicated. Generally, this means an intranet, or possibly groupware such as Lotus Notes, perhaps with special features for easy input of information—some systems for extracting 'know how' from a sales force use the ubiquitous mobile phone as the input medium.
- *Cultural*: the ways in which the organization adapts its reward and recognition systems, and other behavioural norms, to ensure that staff are encouraged in fact, rather than just in abstract, to share their knowledge.
- *Intellectual*: the means by which the knowledge to be managed can be identified—issues of 'content'—and the ways in which it can be represented and organized for subsequent access.

This third aspect is crucial for the success of KM, but is often overlooked in an enthusiasm to get the first two components right.

In practice, pharmaceutical information services are likely to become involved in knowledge management in one of two ways. Some organizations are placing considerable stress on creating 'know-how databases', most commonly based on intranet technology, in an attempt to capture the 'soft' knowledge not usually included in conventional databases. Others focus on systems for the identification of individual expertise—the 'expertise index' or 'electronic yellow pages'—on the basis that the only way to transfer such knowledge is by putting the enquirer in direct contact with the knowledgeable person. These mechanisms are not mutually exclusive, and are in many ways an extension of 'traditional' information management activities.

It is unlikely that interest in KM will continue at its late-'90s level. However, it will have a permanent, and valuable, impact on information management, in focusing attention on a form of knowledge which has largely been ignored in the past.

Knowledge organization

A vital component in the management of information and knowledge is the set of intellectual tools available for the organization of knowledge. Only a brief survey can be given here: fuller accounts are given by Taylor (1999), Aitchison et al (2001), Marcella & Newton (1994) and Marcella & Maltby (2000).

The principle tool for organization of knowledge and information in an electronic environment is the metadata used to describe the records (Dempsey & Heery 1998).

Metadata is information *about* information resources, specifically electronic resources. It can be considered as the digital equivalent of the cataloguing record used in traditional library catalogues. It comprises both a description of the subject of the record, and other descriptive material, e.g. author, physical form, version, date of submission, etc. Knowledge organization is concerned largely with subject description.

Although subject retrieval can be achieved by searching full text, or by assignment of 'free' indexing terms automatically or intellectually, experience suggests that information management benefits from the use of controlled vocabularies for subject description. These are, largely, traditional library / information techniques of classification and indexing.

Strengths of controlled languages are:

- make life easier for the searcher
- control synonyms and near-synonyms
- show broader, narrower and related terms
- provide 'semantic map' of a subject area
- provide descriptive scope notes and homographs for terms
- express concepts elusive in free text
- express broad 'area' concepts missing in free text
- help to overcome syntax problems with devices such as compound terms
- avoid over-indexing, by omitting minor concepts
- can improve both recall and precision
- essential aid in a multi-lingual system
- particularly powerful in numeric / factual systems, where text is not rich.

Controlled vocabularies are divided into those which bring subjects together (systematic or classified vocabularies) and those which bring similar words together (alphabetical arrangements). There are close links between the two forms: most classification schemes will have an alphabetic index, and alphabetically arranged thesauri are always based on a classificatory analysis.

Classification may be applied to:

- knowledge—concepts, expressed in words
- physical things—plants, animals, chemicals
- information artifacts—books, articles etc.

All classifications are artificial. Despite the long search for a 'natural' classification, it must be accepted that all classifications are, to some degree, arbitrary, and are to be judged only by their usefulness in practice.

- Classification shows the relations between concepts; particularly, though not exclusively, hierarchical concepts.
- Classification is a process of categorizing concepts into mutually exclusive sets, by rational principles of division.
- Particular items can rarely be classified absolutely, but rather on the basis of overall similarity.

To be useful, a classification must:

- apply to similar things
- give sets similar in nature and size
- apply consistent criteria for division
- apply one criterion at a time.

Classification has two main purposes:

- physical arrangement of material, e.g. books on library shelves
- retrieval by subject.

The latter may be either by direct retrieval, e.g. from a card catalogue or computer system, or browsing.

Classification is particularly valuable for a broad, browsing approach to retrieval.

There are four main kinds of classification:

- broad categorizations (for browsing and physical arrangement)
- enumerative (hierarchical) classifications (for physical arrangement and retrieval)
- analytico-synthetic (faceted) classifications (for detailed retrieval)
- hypertext and similar classifications (for browsing).

Broad categorizations, useful for browsing and for physical arrangement, are a simple form of classification with little or no hierarchical structure. They are used in several settings: in smaller libraries, where a simple structure with a high degree of browsability is required, or where fiction is a large component of stock; in bookshops; and as an additional search tool in some computerized databases, particularly in the humanities and social sciences. It is feasible for an individual library or information unit to devise its own system of categorization.

Enumerative classifications are used for physical arrangement, particularly in larger libraries, and for subject retrieval. They aim to include (enumerate) all aspects of knowledge within their scope; they are invariably hierarchically arranged, dividing and subdividing knowledge. They are well suited for arranging large volumes of material, especially when a physical arrangement, with a place for each item, is required, and hence are widely used for library classification. They have severe limitations in dealing with very detailed subject description, and with items involving several concepts. They are also unsuitable for rapidly changing subject fields, since they cannot be revised frequently.

Examples are:

- Decimal (Dewey)
- Universal Decimal (UDC)
- National Library of Medicine.

It would not be feasible for an individual library or information unit to create its own enumerative classification, although local modifications are possible.

Analytico-synthetic classifications, generally used for retrieval of detailed subject concepts, are commonly termed faceted classifications. Terminology is grouped into 'facets' of related subjects (hence analytic), from which the classification for any item can be constructed (hence synthetic); these classifications can then cope with new concepts in a way in which enumerative schemes cannot. This type of representation was very popular during the 1950s and '60s for classifying specialized or technical material, but is relatively little used today. However, facet analysis underlies most thesauri, which are still in common use. It would be feasible for a library or information unit to devise a faceted classification scheme, either for its own sake, or as a step to thesaurus construction.

Hypertext and similar classifications allow browsing and navigating among information, either within a single document (micro-hypertext) or within a database (macro-hypertext). To whatever information representation is present (typically full-text) is added a set of hypertext links, joining pieces of information which the analyst considers will be useful for users to browse between. Examples of micro-hypertext are procedure manuals, legal texts etc.

The best known example of macro-hypertext is the worldwide web tool on the internet. Here, the 'classification' is subjective and piecemeal, based on local similarity. An interesting comparison can be made between this form of classification on the world wide web and systems for broad categorization of its material, e.g. the Yahoo subject directory.

Alphabetic term lists are commonly used for information management purposes. Standard lists and thesauri exist for most subject areas, but it is possible for an information unit to construct its own list.

Keyword lists, subject headings may take various forms, but in essence they are simply lists of the terms used for indexing in a particular system. They may show synonyms, and preferred terms, but not usually other relations between terms.

Thesauri are listings of terms with inter-term relations shown. There are various relations which may be used, but the standard set is:

- SY : synonym
- BT : broader term
- NT : narrower term
- RT : related term.

Thesauri were originally devised to deal with the problems of information retrieval from manual systems, e.g. card files, or from early mechanized systems, e.g. punched card sorters. The widespread use of computer systems, with consequent ability to search full text, or a surrogate for it, e.g. titles and abstracts, using natural language free text, has cast some doubt on the need for any form of vocabulary control. Some computerized retrieval systems appear to manage well enough without it. However, experience has shown that some form of vocabulary control, based on subject analysis, is essential for the most effective use of virtually any information retrieval system. Indeed, many advanced information processing systems, including some based on so-called artificial intelligence, have, in effect, had to reinvent the thesaurus.

In general, it may be said that for greatest effectiveness any computerized retrieval system should incorporate both controlled and free-text access, and this is provided in many current systems. Natural language provides precision and exact specificity of current terminology, while the controlled vocabulary links together related terms, for high recall, and may provide devices to improve precision.

There are several published thesauri relevant to pharmaceutical information, including:

- MeSH (National Library of Medicine Medical Subject Headings)
- Emtree (Excerpta Medica)
- Derwent thesaurus
- Martindale
- Pharmline.

Thesauri may be used in three ways for information retrieval:

- for both indexing and searching
- for indexing, but not searching
- for searching, but not indexing.

The first way is still most common. The second and third are becoming more popular to aid end-user searching in computerized retrieval systems.

Information mapping and auditing

Definitions

The definition proposed by the Aslib Information Resources Management Network has become a standard in the UK: a systematic examination of information use, resources and flows, with a verification by reference to both people and existing documents, in order to establish the extent to which they are contributing to an organization's objectives.

Orna (1999) defines what the audit examines as:

- the information an organization holds which can be turned into knowledge by people and applied in their work to meet its objectives
- the resources for making information accessible to those who need to turn it into knowledge
- the ways in which it uses information to further its objectives
- the people who are involved in using information
- the 'tools' it uses for doing things with information
- the criteria it uses to assess the costs and values of information.

These definitions have important implications. The starting point has to be what the organization is trying to do, and what that means about information requirements and use—'what should be'. The process requires asking appropriate questions to find out 'what is'; and the output is the result of comparing the two and interpreting the results (Orna 1999).

Information mapping

Information auditing as just described is comparable to the 'information resource discovery process' described by Burk & Horton (1988) in their *Infomap: A complete guide to discovering corporate information resources*.

This has four main steps:

- preliminary resource inventory—starting from a tentative model of what you expect to encounter
- examination of the cost and value of entities identified in the first step with the aim of getting 'some kind of cost/value ratio . . . even if only rough approximations'
- analysis: examination of the findings from the first two steps to find where resources are distributed, the basic nature of each, the magnitude and location of costs and values. This leads to 'charts and maps' which form springboards for raising questions on management policies, etc. and highlight gaps, overlaps and redundancies
- synthesis: assessment of the quality of identified resources expressed in terms of relative strengths and weaknesses.

Essential resources and support for information auditing

- Support from top management and clear reporting line to top level of decision making via management champion
- people with knowledge, experience, judgement and standing to run it
- time allowance
- guaranteed access to people and documents
- appropriate finance (information auditing need not be a costly business, compared with other expenditures which are accepted without question; for some illuminating figures and comparisons, see the case study of information auditing in Surrey Police, in Orna, 1999).

Senior management need to understand and give commitment to the objectives of the audit, the scope and phasing proposed, the deliverables from the audit, and the resources required. People in the organization who will be affected by the audit need full information about it, the opportunity to ask questions, express anxieties, receive explanations, and a guarantee of taking part in discussing the findings and contributing to decisions. Without that, they will feel threatened and will not contribute their knowledge—to the detriment of the quality and reliability of findings.

Planning – selecting key areas for projects

The safest and most productive way of running an information audit is through a series of projects; it allows learning on the job with minimal risks, and gives the chance of 'quick wins' that gain support for the process. The best areas are those where information has high strategic importance and/or potential for adding value; a project area should have a clear boundary and not be too big; and it should be tackled by people who are information-aware and/or have a problem they really want to crack.

Pharmaceutical example

Following structural changes in the pharmaceutical company mentioned earlier, which resulted from a study of how its investment in IT was supporting the business, the company set up two auditing projects:

- analysis of documents it produced for regulatory submissions, to identify the actual and potential information sources and the way information was used in submissions
- investigation of how systems development related to company information needs and to researchers' work tasks (there was some evidence that it was ad hoc and one-off, without meaningful criteria for priorities).

Who does it and who do they need to talk to?

Varying views have been expressed on this; the current consensus is probably that the audit should be managed and controlled from inside the organization, with the main work done by the organization's staff—drawing on appropriate internal and external expertise and support. The core audit management team needs people of good standing, with strategic knowledge of the organization and ability to interact with others. Project management groups should involve those close to the project area.

The main groups of people with whom information auditors need to talk are: the 'guardians' responsible for managing specific kinds of information on behalf of the organization (and the managers to whom they are answerable); and the stakeholders—people who need particular kinds of information in their work, and therefore have a legitimate interest in how it is managed.

Methods

There is no single best method of information auditing. A variety of methods can be successfully used—the key lies in choosing them to match the nature of the organization and the project in hand. They include: analysis of documents and databases; observation of people carrying out information tasks and trying out tasks for oneself; structured interviews; cross functional working groups; questionnaires; visual representations; soft systems analysis. Software support for some of these methods is available; for examples, and for further description of the methods summarized above, see the case studies in Orna (1999). A survey of information mapping and auditing methods, including pharmaceutical examples, such as those carried out by one of the authors of this chapter (DB) at Pfizer Central Research, is given by Ellis et al (1993). Huotari (1995), Trzan-Herman & Kiauta (1996), and Bawden et al (2000) give further examples of information auditing and mapping in pharmaceutical information services.

Pharmaceutical example

Methods used in the exemplar pharmaceutical company for the projects listed above included:

- cross-functional and cross-discipline groups for exchange of ideas

- user workshops to formulate problems, run by users with systems/IT specialists as a knowledge resource, and a 'management champion' to hold the ring
- managers' workshops, to look at the problems identified by user workshops, selected the agenda of the next stages. The output consisted of a list of all systems for which users had stated requirement; and the facts on document architecture.

Key areas

In any audit project, the key areas are:

- information resources
- guardians and stakeholders
- information flow and interactions
- systems and technology supporting information use
- how the cost-effectiveness of information is assessed.

A lot of preparation time needs to go into deciding the questions to ask and how to ask them, trying them out to ensure that they are unambiguous, and making sure that all the people concerned in finding the answers agree about what they are doing.

While the audit is in progress, the audit team needs to meet frequently, to exchange news of what they are finding, resolve unexpected problems, note points that look likely to require recommendations for action.

Interpreting the findings—matching what is with what should be

The heart of information auditing is matching 'what is' with 'what should be' to identify good and bad matches in areas where information is of high strategic importance. The picture of where there is convergence or divergence between the two makes the foundation for meaningful presentation of results, and proposals for action.

Pharmaceutical example

Key findings from the project mentioned above were:

- a variety of PCs and software were in use and users were often without any support
- there was no standardization on word-processing software
- end-user computing projects were going on in many locations without any overall evaluation and coordination
- there were no agreed priority criteria for ranking user requests for professionally developed systems to support research, and nobody had responsibility for coordinating these requests
- incompatible equipment slowed data transfer
- there were no standards for content and layout of internal documents
- there were organizational problems in getting data from support departments.

Actions recommended:

- selection of integrated end-user system development kit
- corporate standards for systems development, and adoption of single word-processing standard throughout company
- set of critical success factors based on business objectives to be used as criteria for allocating priority among requests for systems development
- working party on how reports were compiled, with remit of defining standards
- continued monitoring by 'management champion' and presentation of findings to the company's board.

This particular example emphasizes IT and information system aspects. These are important in information management as a whole, and indeed form the basis for any IM strategy;

hence it is vital that information professionals are familiar with them, and are involved along with IT staff in their selection and implementation. They can also provide their own specific contribution to IM strategy development, based on an in-depth understanding of the content of information sources, and their relevance to users and to the organization , and on the intellectual techniques of information organization and retrieval; the semantic and pragmatic aspects noted above.

After the audit

Presentation of findings and recommendations for action should flow without break into decisions, and decisions into action. Action plans should aim for:

- essential changes to avoid immediate threats
- quick benefits in key areas to keep up momentum, maintain commitment to change
- maintaining communication links established during the audit
- definitive statement of organizational information policy
- developing an organizational information strategy in the project area
- setting appropriate criteria for monitoring and evaluating changes as implemented
- making the information audit into a regular exercise
- regular reporting on information developments at the top level, to feed into business strategy development
- a start on assessing the cost-effectiveness of information use and its contribution to value of organization's assets.

Developing information policy and strategy

Definitions

An organizational information policy is founded on an organization's overall objectives, and priorities within them, and defines several aspects at a general level (Orna 1999):

- the objectives of information use in the organization, and the priorities among them
- what 'information' means in the context of what the organization is in business for
- the principles on which it will manage information
- principles for the use of human resources in managing information
- principles for the use of technology to support information management
- the principles it will apply in relation to establishing the cost-effectiveness of information and knowledge.

An organizational information strategy is the detailed expression of information policy in terms of objectives, targets, and actions to achieve them, for a defined period ahead. It provides the framework for the management of information and, supported by appropriate systems and technology, can be the 'engine' for maintaining, managing and applying the organization's information resources. It supports the organization's essential knowledge base.

Information systems/IT strategy depends on what information the organization needs, and how it needs to use it. It deals with applications software and infrastructure to support information management.

Distinctions

Information policy is at the level of principles, embodied in a short statement which can be developed at one go, and is meant to last. It can be developed in outline form as part of the preparation for an information audit, and refined in the light of the findings.

Information strategy is the basis for action for a given period. It is reviewed at frequent intervals, and can be developed and implemented in stages.

What a policy should cover

To start with, there should be a statement of the basic obligations of employees and of the organization in respect of information That should be followed by a simple statement of the principles the organization will follow in managing information, emphasizing those elements which a preliminary analysis and/or information audit has shown to be critical for the organization.

Essential commitments include:

- defining information in organizational terms
- proper management and safeguarding of information resources
- a coordinated overview of total resources
- promotion of essential information interchanges
- appropriate systems/IT infrastructure
- ethical use of knowledge and information
- maximum openness of access
- application of reliable means of assessing the costs of information and its value contribution to achieving objectives
- appropriate human and financial resources.

Information policy as foundation for information strategy

The process of 'selling' an information policy upwards, and especially outwards, makes the best foundation for developing an information strategy. It involves getting information management written into corporate objectives and encouraging people to buy into information strategy.

Developing and using information strategy

The process of question asking and answering described above (see pp. 39–41), and of comparing 'what is' with 'what should be' in information auditing provides the material for information strategy development. The developers should include: managers of all kinds of information resources, managers of information systems/IT, representative stakeholders in information resources, and managers responsible for corporate strategy. The process needs the same kind of resources as information auditing.

Focal points for development

As with information auditing, a phased approach to strategy development offers learning potential, combined with low risk and the chance of quick wins. Focal points: the organization's strengths, unique features, core competencies, survival essentials (including things it is not very good at, and areas of risk), potential for innovation.

Pharmaceutical example

The key points for action identified in the example of the pharmaceutical company suggest these focal points for information strategy development:

- *standards development*: corporate standards for systems development and software; standards for compilation and presentation of reports for regulatory submissions
- *critical success factors*: extension of the process developed for allocating priorities in systems development to other key business areas

Bristol-Myers Squibb Pharmaceuticals Ltd
Medical Information Enquiry

UK Log No.

Date & Time ─────────────────── **Received By** ───────────────

Product
(Trade/Generic) ──────────────────

Customer Name ─────────────────

Deadline
(Date) ───────────────────────────

Customer Address ──────────────

Representative ────────────────

Mobile Number ─────────────────

Post Code ──────────────
(compulsory)

Customer Status
☐ Hospital Doctor   ☐ Hospital Pharmacist   ☐ Nurse
☐ General   ☐ Community Pharmacist   ☐ Internal
   Practitioner
☐ Other (specify) ───────────────

Telephone
(Ext/Page) ────────────────

Fax ─────────────────────

Enquiry Details

───────────────────────────────────────
───────────────────────────────────────
───────────────────────────────────────
───────────────────────────────────────
───────────────────────────────────────
───────────────────────────────────────
───────────────────────────────────────
───────────────────────────────────────
───────────────────────────────────────
───────────────────────────────────────
───────────────────────────────────────
───────────────────────────────────────
───────────────────────────────────────

ADE
Sex
Age
Other Medication

Dosage/Duration

Hospitalisation

Summary/Response

───────────────────────────────────────
───────────────────────────────────────
───────────────────────────────────────
───────────────────────────────────────
───────────────────────────────────────
───────────────────────────────────────
───────────────────────────────────────
───────────────────────────────────────
───────────────────────────────────────
───────────────────────────────────────
───────────────────────────────────────
───────────────────────────────────────
───────────────────────────────────────
───────────────────────────────────────

Information Sources
☐ Standard Letter
☐ SPC
☐ PIL
☐ Internal Database
☐ On-Line Search
☐ Reference Text
☐ Other Dept
   (specify) ─────────
☐ Other
   (specify) ─────────

Attempts to call back:

Reply sent via: ☐ Telephone   ☐ Letter   ☐ Email   ☐ Fax   ☐ Personal

Actioned By: ───────── **Date Completed** ───────── **Time Taken (mins)** ─────────

Figure 5.1   *Bristol-Myers Squibb Pharmaceuticals Ltd Medical Information Enquiry Form*

The information professional should always ask the question 'does anyone else need to know about this enquiry?' or 'would someone else be better qualified to provide an answer?' and act accordingly.

Step 4—Obtain background information

This step involves establishing the nature and circumstances of the enquiry with the aim of gaining a better understanding of it. The information professional will thus be able to provide a more useful and relevant response.

In many cases customers find it difficult to express their true information needs. Sometimes it may be that their knowledge of the subject is limited and they are not sure how to ask the right question. Kirkwood (1996) describes a survey of drug information questions handled by the Drug Information service at the Medical College of Virginia hospitals. The survey was conducted over a 6-month period and showed that for 85% of enquiries received, the ultimate question researched was significantly different from the original question. In these cases the customer was satisfied with the final response received.

A key part of the information professional's job is to determine whether the question that the customer has asked fully represents what he or she wants to know. This can be done by finding out why the information is needed and considering what other information may be relevant. It is important not to assume anything, to check details and ask questions. The aim is to develop a clear picture of what the real enquiry is—Kirkwood (1996) terms this the 'ultimate question'. Ascione et al (1994) describe this as transforming the original query into the 'real question'.

If the information professional can truly answer the question 'why is this customer asking for this information?' then adequate background information has been obtained.

For enquiries involving the treatment of a specific patient the following information should be obtained:

- patient details
- medical history
- function of major body systems, e.g. renal, hepatic, cardiovascular
- drug history
- other relevant information.

Table 5.1 provides a guide to additional questions that may need to be asked to obtain background information for different enquiry classifications.

It is important to balance the need for background information with the customer's and the information professional's time. Only appropriate and relevant questions should be asked. The information professional should establish a dialogue with the customer to obtain the necessary details.

Obtaining background information may be an underestimated skill. Kirkwood (1996) describes an anecdotal observation suggesting that there is a significant loss of skill if an information professional is absent from handling enquiries for more than eight consecutive weeks.

Step 5—Reformulate and understand the real enquiry

Once background information has been collected the information professional is in a position to confirm the true enquiry before developing a search strategy to find the relevant information to answer the enquiry. It is important to establish if the customer has searched any information sources already.

The information professional needs to ensure that there is a very clear understanding of exactly what answer needs to be found. Summarizing the enquiry back to the customer should ensure that both the customer and the information professional are clear about the question that is going to be answered.

Enquiry classification	Additional questions
Adverse drug reaction	What are the signs and symptoms of the possible reaction?
	What is the duration and severity of the reaction?
	What is the time relationship between drug administration and the reaction?
	What is the current medical status of the patient?
	What other medications is the patient taking?
	What is the patient's age, weight/body surface area, sex and race?
	Why was the patient receiving the drug?
	What other disease conditions does the patient have?
	What is the renal and hepatic function of the patient?
	Has the patient experienced this adverse reaction before?
	Was the suspected drug ever administered before?
	Why was it discontinued?
Compatibility/stability	What are fluid volume or electrolyte restrictions?
	What are the available routes of administration?
	What is the indication for treatment?
	What is the site and type of drug contact (IV administration set, syringe, bottle, device, glass or PVC)?
	What is the suspected time of contact?
	What is the IV solution and what are the additives?
	What are the storage conditions?
	What are the doses, concentrations and volumes of all medications?
Dosage	What is the indication for treatment?
	What is the patient's body weight/body surface area?
	What is the diagnosis of the patient and the indication for drug use?
	What is the patient's age, sex and race?
	What is the patient's renal and liver function?
	What is the route of administration?
	What other drugs are being taken?
	What other disease conditions does the patient have?
	Is the patient on a restricted fluid or sodium intake which may affect how a drug is administered?
Drug interactions	Has the enquiry been made to avoid an interaction or to investigate a suspected interaction?
	What is the suspected interaction?
	What drugs is the patient taking?
	What are the doses, duration and administration timings of each of the drugs?
	Is drug-drug interference suspected?
	Is drug-food interference suspected?
	Is drug-laboratory test interference suspected?
	What other disease conditions does the patient have?
Clinical use/drug choice	What is the indication for treatment?
	What is the patient's age, sex, race and weight/body surface area?
	What are the patient's renal and hepatic functions?
	Is the patient taking any other medications?
	What are the current medical problems that may be affected by the drug?
Identification of a drug	What is the reason for the enquiry—large amount ingested, foreign product, equivalent needed?

Table 5.1 *Additional questions to obtain background information*

	What are the dosage form and appearance (size, shape, identifying marks, letters, numbers)? What is the country of origin of the drug? What are the drug's trade and generic names? What is the spelling of the drug's names? What is the drug thought to be used to treat? What is the source of information about the drug?
Pharmacokinetics	What are the possible routes of drug administration for the patient? What is the hepatic and renal function of the patient? What is the dosing history for the patient? Are body fluid drug levels available and what is their relationship to dosage form administered and time since last dose? What is the patient's age, sex, race and weight/body surface area? Why is the patient being treated and what is the severity of the illness? What other disease conditions does the patient have?
Pregnancy	Did the patient take the drug? Is the patient pregnant or planning to become pregnant? What is the dose, route, frequency and duration of treatment? What trimester of pregnancy is the patient in? Why is the drug to be given? What is the patient's age, weight/body surface area?
Lactation	Is the patient breastfeeding? Was the baby exposed to the drug? What are the clinical signs/symptoms in the breastfed baby? What are the time course and sequence of events? What is the dose, duration and frequency of dosing?
Teratogenicity	Was the fetus exposed to the drug? Did the drug possibly cause an abnormality in the child? What are the dose, frequency, route and duration of therapy? What are the clinical manifestations? What are the time course and sequence of events?
Toxicology	What was the amount of drug ingested? Were other medications ingested? When was the drug ingested? Were other substances ingested, e.g. alcohol, attempted remedies? What was the route of administration or exposure? Does the patient's history indicate if signs or symptoms are developing? What was done to treat the patient? What is the patient's age, sex, race, weight/body surface area?

Step 6—Agree the time frame

The expected time frame must be discussed with the customer. This may need to be negotiated based on the customer's needs and a realistic assessment of the time it will take to answer the enquiry. The depth and format of the response should also be agreed.

It is critical to contact the customer within the time agreed. Updates on progress should be given if necessary. The information professional must provide a full response by the agreed deadline or, at a minimum, some preliminary feedback.

Step 7—Search for relevant information

Once the true enquiry has been clarified, the search for relevant information can begin.

The use and choice of information sources is covered in more detail later in this chapter.

The essence of an effective search is that it is conducted in a logical manner, so that relevant information is identified in a timely way. An efficient and effective search is a cheaper search.

Step 8—Analyse and evaluate the information

The analysis and evaluation of information is covered in more detail in Chapter 6.

The information collected in the search needs to be collated and reviewed. The quality of each piece of information should be assessed objectively and the parts which are relevant to the enquiry should be highlighted. Usually one piece of information does not fully answer the question—further assessment and synthesis of additional information is needed to reach a conclusion.

Step 9—Formulate a response

The information professional needs to have in mind what is required for the reply, provide relevant information and organize it so that it really answers the true question.

A useful approach to take is to:

- list the information sources searched
- write down statements from the sources that are relevant to the answer
- prepare a summary of the relevant information
- include detailed information if necessary
- be prepared for additional questions from the customer.

The response should be organized and logical and all information sources should be clearly documented. It should be succinct but comprehensive enough to answer the question.

The information professional has to be able to adapt responses to suit the needs of different customers. Patients may require a simple explanation of a topic whereas a hospital consultant might need a fully documented review of a subject supported by a literature search.

Step 10—Communicate the response

Good verbal communication skills are essential for providing the ideal response to a customer. Deciding whether the information should be provided in writing or orally is also important—assessing the approach that is most likely to result in the customer having a clear understanding of the response.

If no clear answer is found then it is important to explain the information sources that were used. The customer should feel confident that the question was thoroughly researched even though no information to answer the question was found.

Step 11—Follow up

Actively following up the responses to enquiries helps to check the quality and appropriateness of the information. A telephone call to discuss how useful the response to the enquiry was to the customer and the customer's views of the quality of the service is an effective way of following up enquiries. This approach can be quite time-consuming and an alternative method is to send the customer a brief questionnaire or reply-paid card to ask for the customer's assessment of the response and how the enquiry was handled. This is all part of a professional approach to handling customer enquiries and good customer service.

Follow-up enables the information professional to find out:

- was the right question asked and the right answer given?
- was it clear and understood?
- what impact did it have on patient care, how was the information used?
- can further assistance be given?

Information sources

The selection of appropriate information sources is an important step in the process of providing answers to customers' enquiries. Handling enquiries effectively requires a sound knowledge of the types of information sources available, with an understanding of their pros and cons and suitability for different subjects.

Types of information sources

Information sources have traditionally been described in three categories—primary, secondary and tertiary. This categorization is still useful as a means of classifying different sources and determining at which stage of the enquiry handling process they are likely to be most appropriate.

Primary information sources are those which include original research and ideas, or case reports. Examples of primary information sources are scientific journals, such as the *British Medical Journal* and *Lancet*. Secondary information sources include abstracting or indexing services and online databases, examples include Medline and Embase. These sources provide a means of access to the primary literature. Reference texts which contain reviews and overviews of topics are examples of tertiary information sources. Chapter 2 covers the different types of information sources in more detail.

The use of computerized information sources is an essential part of the information professional's role. The efficient and effective use of these sources demands a great deal of skill and knowledge. An understanding of the types of information source, the selection of appropriate databases, awareness of costs and a systematic approach are essential in the effective use of computerized sources.

The internet is an increasingly important source of information and is now a core resource for the information professional. All three types of information source (primary, secondary and tertiary) can be found on the internet. It is particularly useful for news stories and current information. One of the most important considerations in using the internet as an information source is being aware of the source of the information and making a judgement about its quality.

Other information sources include company bibliographic databases, internal company reports and expert networks.

Selecting information sources

The best approach to take in using information sources for handling customer enquiries is to start with generalized tertiary sources and move through secondary sources towards more specific primary information sources. This approach enables the information professional to move from getting a clear overview of the subject to identifying specific information relevant to the question the customer has asked.

General information ⸻⟶ Specific information

Using this approach effectively demands good knowledge of the content of each of the information sources as well as the ability to search the resource. The information professional is then able to prioritize available resources on the basis of how likely they are to contain relevant information. This forms a search strategy for utilizing the different information sources that are available. The information professional needs to be prepared to adjust and refine this strategy during the search, according to the information that is found.

Primary information sources provide the most detailed information but it may be difficult to search them for specific data. In-house bibliographic databases with additional specific indexing are used by pharmaceutical companies to facilitate searching the primary literature. It is important to use the original source wherever possible as data may be misinterpreted by other authors. For example, a review article may provide a useful summary of a topic but the original studies referenced in the review article should be evaluated to ensure that the data relevant to the enquiry are accurately interpreted.

Secondary information sources make it easier to retrieve information but are less current due to the time delay in abstracting and indexing the primary literature.

Tertiary sources are more limited as they may reflect the author's selection of the data available and are less current. They are very practical as specialized resources are available for handling different types of enquiry. For example, textbooks on drug interactions provide a very good starting point for enquiries on drug-drug and drug-food interactions.

Another factor that will determine which information sources are used is the time frame available to provide a response. Where limited time is available a thorough search of all information sources will not be possible and prioritization of the most relevant sources is critical.

The final choice of information sources to use for an individual enquiry will depend on:

- classification of enquiry
- type of customer
- time frame
- depth of response required
- costs incurred in using sources.

Citing information sources

There are a number of different methods used for citing information sources in written documents. This book uses the Ciba alphabetical system in which authors are cited in the text by name and year of publication. The format of reference lists is also defined in this system, references being listed in alphabetical order. The order of items in a journal reference using the Ciba alphabetical system is:

- author name(s) and initials
- year of publication
- title of reference
- title of journal
- volume number
- issue number
- page range.

An alternative system is the Ciba numerical system where references in the text are referred to using superscript numerals. Reference lists present the references in numerical order.

The Vancouver style is also widely used. References in the text are cited with superscript numerals with reference lists being presented in numerical order. The formatting of citations in the reference list is different from that of the Ciba system. The order of items in a reference in the Vancouver system is:

- author name(s) and initials
- title of reference

- title of journal
- year of publication
- volume number
- issue number
- page range.

The choice of referencing system is not important. What is important is that references are cited using one system and that system is applied consistently and accurately so that the reader can easily find a reference source.

Recommended information sources

Several authors and professional organizations have provided guides to the most appropriate information sources for handling drug information enquiries (Ascione et al 1994, Malone et al 1996, Millares 1998). These guides act as useful training resources to the new information professional and help in familiarization with relevant information sources. They also act as guidance to departments on appropriate resource levels for providing a service of adequate quality.

AIOPI has created a list of key information sources for medical information departments in the pharmaceutical industry (Association of Information Officers in the Pharmaceutical Industry, 1999). The UK Drug Information Pharmacists Group also gives guidance on minimum information sources for Drug Information departments in the UK National Health Service (Judd, 1997).

Departmental information sources

The majority of medical information departments will have their own sources of information, such as question and answer databases and standard responses. These sources serve a number of important purposes:

- records of customer enquiries handled by the department—enabling retrieval of past enquiries
- single source of information on a specific topic—ensuring consistency of responses
- responses to frequently asked questions—ensuring that a quick response can be provided to customers.

These departmental information sources help the information professional to satisfy the customer's need for an efficient and timely service and also help in ensuring a consistent quality of information. It is important to ensure that a ready prepared information summary is relevant to the question that the customer has asked and will be an appropriate response. The ability of the information professional to judge the relevance of a response to the customer's information need is critical. Where necessary a decision to tailor the response to address exactly what the customer wants to know will be required. This is an important aspect of providing quality customer service. The temptation to provide an answer quickly should be resisted if the answer does not fully address the needs of the customer.

Communication skills

The effective handling of customer enquiries requires good communication skills to ensure that the customer's information need is clearly established and that the response is delivered effectively and is understood by the customer.

Key skills that are required include listening, questioning, written and oral communications.

Listening skills

Good listening skills are fundamental to providing an effective information service, particularly when customer enquiries are received by telephone where verbal communication is the only method available.

Questioning skills

Effective use of questioning is critical in receiving an enquiry to ensure that the real needs of the customer are uncovered and the necessary background information is obtained.

The choice of question and the way in which it is asked is important. As Mackay (1980) points out, success in using questioning 'depends on asking the right questions and accurately assessing the responses in order to make the right decisions.' Mackay (1980) also notes that 'once a question is asked, the questioner becomes the listener'. This is further reinforcement of the importance of good listening skills.

Oral communication

The ability to explain information and clarify a response is a fundamental aspect of the role of an information professional.

Written communication

Communicating information clearly in a written form is becoming increasingly important as technological developments, such as fax, email, and the internet have increased the demand for written confirmation of responses to enquiries. Although the majority of enquiries received by a medical information department are received by telephone, an increasing proportion of customers request written information in response.

Cutts (1995) describes Plain English as 'the writing and setting out of essential information in a way that gives a co-operative, motivated person a good chance of understanding the document at first reading, and in the same sense that the writer meant it to be understood.' This is a good way of describing the ideal written response from an information professional.

Goddard (1998) provides a practical guide to informative writing—which he describes as writing which is intended to inform others, rather than persuasive writing (intended to impress or persuade others) or creative writing (intended to create an effect). He advocates use of three principal techniques—planning, writing and revising. The importance of revising is stressed to ensure that the final document is checked and improved.

It is beyond the scope of this book to provide detailed coverage of communication skills. Further reading sources on these topics are provided at the end of the chapter.

Customer care

Many of the concepts described earlier in this chapter are aspects of good customer care. Forsyth (1997) describes customers as having three overriding requirements:

- prompt service
- efficient service
- courteous service.

These requirements mean that information professionals need to be available at the right time for their customers, to treat their customers courteously and as individuals, to have relevant information to hand and to provide explanations clearly.

Bee & Bee (1995) stress the importance of using the term customer to apply to all users of a service, whether they are 'external customers' outside an organization or 'internal customers' within the organization. They point out that the quality of customer care provided to all customers is important and that successful organizations operate as though their colleagues are important customers.

Bee & Bee (1995) define four crucial elements in delivering quality customer care:

- appropriateness—does the service meet the customer's needs?
- consistency/reliability—is the service of the required standard all the time?
- timeliness—is the service provided when the customer needs it and within an appropriate time period?
- satisfying—does the way the service is provided ensure that it is a good experience for the customer, is it friendly and helpful, does it show interest/concern?

An important aspect of any pharmaceutical information service must be providing high quality customer care. Measuring the quality of the service should form part of the ongoing evaluation of the service. The measurement of information services is covered in more detail in Chapters 7, 8, 9 and 10.

As Cook (1997) explains, good customer service is meeting customers' expectations whereas excellent customer service means exceeding their expectations. Information services should be striving for excellence.

Conclusion

The provision of information is one of the critical roles of a pharmaceutical information professional.

IT developments have facilitated the use of different sources of information and new approaches have eliminated human interaction altogether, e.g. internet sites, recorded helplines. However, interpersonal interaction is critical to the effective provision of information. The skills of the information professional are essential in clarifying the true enquiry that the customer wants to have answered. The enquiry handling process requires the application of knowledge and judgement. It also demands the analysis and evaluation of information to provide the customer with the solution to his or her problem.

Customer care should be at the heart of every pharmaceutical information service—striving for excellence and aiming to provide the right information to the right customer at the right time.

References and Further Reading

Adair J 1997 Decision making and problem solving. Institute of Personnel and Development, London

Ascione F J, Manifold C C, Parenti M A 1994 Principles of drug information and scientific literature evaluation. Drug Intelligence Publications, Hamilton, USA

Association of Information Officers in the Pharmaceutical Industry (AIOPI) 1999 UK guidelines on standards for medical information departments. www.aiopi.org.uk

Association of Information Officers in the Pharmaceutical Industry (AIOPI) 1999 Recommended books for medical information departments. www.aiopi.org.uk

Bee F, Bee R 1995 Customer care. Institute of Personnel and Development, London

Cook S 1997 Customer care 2nd edn. Kogan Page, London

Cutts M 1995 The Plain English Guide. Oxford University Press, Oxford

Forsyth P 1997 Telephone skills. Institute of Personnel and Development, London

Galt K A 1994 Analyzing and recording a drug information request, module 1, drug information clinical skills program. American Society of Hospital Pharmacists, Bethesda, USA

Galt K A, Calis K A, Turcasso N M 1994 Preparing a drug information response, module 3, drug information clinical skills program. American Society of Hospital Pharmacists, Bethesda, USA

Goddard K 1998 Informative writing, 2nd edn. Cassell London

Judd A 1997 UK drug information manual 4th edn. UK Drug Information Pharmacists Group (available from Drugs and Poisons Information Service, The General Infirmary, Great George Street, Leeds LS1 3EX, UK)

Kirkwood C F 1996 Modified systematic approach to answering questions. In: Malone P M, Mosdell K W, Kier K L, et al (eds) Drug information: a guide for pharmacists. Appleton and Lange, Stamford, Connecticut

Kneeland S 1999 Solving problems. How To Books, Oxford

Mackay I 1984 Listening skills. Institute of Personnel and Development, London

Mackay I 1980 Asking questions. Institute of Personnel and Development, London

Malone P M, Mosdell K W, Kier K L, et al 1996 Drug information: a guide for pharmacists. Appleton and Lange, Stamford, Connecticut

Millares M 1998 Applied drug information: strategies for information management. Applied Therapeutics, Vancouver

Partridge E 1965 Usage and abusage. Guild Publishing, London

The Oxford Guide to English Usage 2nd edn, 1993 Oxford University Press, Oxford

The Oxford Dictionary of English Grammar 2nd edn, 1993 Oxford University Press, Oxford

Smith G H, Norton L L, Ferrill M H 1994 Evaluating drug literature, module 2, drug information clinical skills program. American Society of Hospital Pharmacists, Bethesda, USA

Watanabe A S, McCart G, Shimomura S, et al 1975 Systematic approach to drug information requests. American Journal of Hospital Pharmacy 32: 1282–1285

Watanabe A S, Conner C S 1978 Principles of drug information services. Drug Intelligence Publications, Hamilton, USA

Chapter 6

Analysing and evaluating information

Frank N Leach

Introduction

In the context of the present chapter, the analysis and evaluation of information is likely to relate to published reports of clinical drug trials, bulletins and/or overviews, journal editorials, promotional material from pharmaceutical companies, the content of discussions with pharmaceutical company representatives, or material obtained from websites.

Evaluation of clinical trial reports will be of particular importance to many readers of this book. Fortunately, the contemporary student of the statistical and methodological aspects of the clinical drug trial has an ample choice of reference material from which to choose, most of it written by very experienced professionals who have a firm grasp of their subject. A plethora of statistical textbooks are available and excellent articles appear from time to time in the leading medical journals. There seemed little point, therefore, in attempting, within this chapter, merely to duplicate or summarize such material. Furthermore, since the present volume is primarily a book for drug information specialists (including pharmacists), I deemed it preferable to attempt an overview of the information evaluation process from their perspective. I have, therefore, based my discussion on my experiences as an erstwhile drug information pharmacist and as tutor to members of the pharmacy, medical, nursing and other professions on the topic of critical evaluation.

A chance invitation, several decades ago, to present an evening lecture on this theme imposed an urgent familiarity with the fundamentals and complexities of the clinical trial process and the related mysteries of statistics. Membership of several ethics committees, both local and multicentre, has intensified my interest in the phenomenon of clinical drug investigation and I have gained much from the observations and comments of fellow committee members, one of whom is a professional statistician.

In my experience, it was not so long ago that pharmacists would often question the propriety of critical evaluation, or their ability to undertake such evaluation, especially when such an exercise was applied to the clinical research output of their medical colleagues. I suspect that such sentiments may linger in some quarters but it now seems almost superfluous to question the relevance of information evaluation skills to the pharmacist or other drug information practitioner. Even the routine process of answering drug-related inquiries, involving the consultation of reference sources, requires a critical assessment of the reliability of such sources.

The medico-legal implications are obvious. Membership of drug and therapeutics committees will impose the need to carefully assess requests for new drugs (and occasionally novel uses for existing drugs), as well as the data on which such requests might be based, and will often require the defence of such assessment. For those involved in preparing drug-related bulletins, bland acceptance of the contents of clinical trial reports or, worse still, the summaries of such reports, may compromise an otherwise balanced appraisal.

Discussions with drug representatives will be enlivened and rendered more productive, when claims for drug products can be challenged or when the inevitable graphs, statistics and other stock in trade of the marketing departments, are brought under scrutiny. Very frequently, the claims made for a drug may hang on a pivotal paper, which may also be the means by which it attains its product licence. Rigorous dissection of such key evidence may often prove critical in formulating guidelines for purchasers and managers. Those elected to serve on ethics committees will usually find that the methodology of proposed investigations will receive as much attention as factors relevant to the safety and dignity of trial participants. The routine inclusion of statisticians as members of the relatively novel multicentre research ethics committees (MRECs) reflects this significant change in attitudes. Trials which are faulty in design and which are, therefore, incapable of providing a satisfactory outcome are deemed unethical since they are deemed to waste resources and to place trial participants at needless risk and inconvenience.

One factor, which probably more than any other has emphasized the importance of critical information appraisal, has been the emergence of an evidence-based medicine culture. This advocates systematic and rigorous evaluation of evidence in all branches of medicine towards a goal of standard guidelines for disease treatment. The emergence of various advisory centres, such as the UK's National Prescribing Centre and National Institute for Clinical Excellence is a further reflection of this trend. It could be argued that the availability of such centres and of the advice which they provide might obviate the need for personal evaluation skills but, at present, this seems unlikely. Today's health professional is sufficiently inundated with drug information in a wide variety of guises to justify the development of a critical, rather than cynical, disposition.

The evolution of the randomized, double-blind, controlled trial

At present, the randomized, double-blind, controlled trial (RCT) is generally regarded as the gold standard method of evaluation of drugs and other forms of treatment or intervention.

Worthy though it might be, the RCT is not an infallible tool and an essential adjunct to its use is adequate recognition of its potential weaknesses. One of the most important of these is the phenomenon of biological variability. Human beings have remarkable diversity in their response to drugs and in their propensity to drug-related adverse effects, to mention but two examples. The potent interaction between mental state and disease response has been more than amply demonstrated; the strong placebo response seen in certain disorders is one example of such an effect. For reasons such as these, unthinking acceptance of the outcome of clinical trials, especially in response to impressive statistical P values, is unwise. These considerations are not cause for despondency. Use of clinical trials has undoubtedly been a significant factor in medical progress and is endorsed by many decades of use.

One of the earliest exponents of the clinical drug trial was Fibiger (1898), who used it successfully to assess the value of serum treatment for diphtheria. Fibiger attempted a crude, but well-intentioned, method of randomization, which involved allocation of treatment (or no treatment) according to the day of hospital admission, as a means of avoiding selection bias. It is commonly held that the first properly randomized controlled trial was that of the UK Medical Research Council, in assessing the efficacy of streptomycin in the treatment of pulmonary tuberculosis (Medical Research Council 1948). The MRC tuberculosis trial was actually predated by a controlled trial of immunization against whooping cough, the results of which were not, however, published until 1951 (Medical Research Council 1951). The tuberculosis trial compared treatment with streptomycin combined with bed rest against bed rest alone. The results, at least in the view of the authors, left no room for doubt that streptomycin dramatically reduced both mortality and radiological evidence of tuberculosis infection. Clearly, albeit with the wisdom of hindsight, there were patients in this study whose lives could have been saved by streptomycin, a consideration which raises important ethical issues. The recognition by doctors and others of the ethical aspects of clinical research, including drug trials, has borne fruit in the network of ethics committees mentioned above.

The quality of clinical trials

With gradual acceptance of the RCT as the key tool of drug assessment, attention has increasingly focused on the quality of trial reports. One of the main reasons for this has been the emphasis on trials to detect differences between active drugs, where such differences, although small, may be clinically significant. It is frequently reiterated, for example, that a difference of as little as 10% in efficacy between two drugs may have important patient-care implications, especially in the context of serious and life-threatening conditions. To detect such a difference requires carefully tuned and scientifically robust studies, far more so than when a new drug is compared with a pharmacologically inactive placebo.

A classic initiative in the area of clinical trial report evaluation, was the publication of a study by Lionel & Herxheimer (1970). This examined, on the basis of a number of defined criteria, the quality of published clinical trial reports in a number of leading medical journals. The outcome of the study was disturbing, showing that approximately one third of the sample of reports were unacceptable as sources of information, in having serious defects in methodology and/or analysis. Reliance on such reports to define patient treatment might have put patients at risk. The checklist of Lionel & Herxheimer remains worthy of inspection, in spite of being partly outdated by the more recent introduction of meta-analysis and increasingly sophisticated means of statistical analysis. Much more recently, the CONSORT statement (Begg et al 1996) has listed 21 key items that should be included in clinical trials. This is obligatory reading for every student of this topic although its approach has not escaped criticism (Meade et al 1997). Views have been expressed that evidence-based medicine, excellent though it might be, cannot provide all the answers and that it might even threaten the art of patient care (Naylor 1995).

Scope of this chapter

In gathering my thoughts for an evaluation strategy, I decided that a good starting point would be a dissection of a clinical trial report. We can then consider, in more detail, some specific issues such as trial subject, drug use and design. It is impossible to avoid mention of the statistical aspects of the RCT and, in particular, the use of meta-analysis but this section is deliberately superficial. Finally, it is important to consider briefly the area of drug promotional material and interaction with the drug representative. I have studiously avoided use of any mathematical formulae or detailed exposition of individual statistical tests. This aversion springs from some bad personal experiences as a recipient of a series of statistics lectures, which proved so obscure that I was deluded into thinking that the null hypothesis was the brainchild of a mathematician, Dr Null. I have also tried to avoid the distraction of too many reference citations.

A broad evaluation of a clinical trial report

Prior to immersion in the finer points of evaluation, we need to consider the broad overview of a clinical trial report. In many ways, the process is akin to the interaction between a patient and a doctor. The latter will usually preface any detailed examinations or tests with a general assessment in order to gain an impression of the patient's general state of health. Similarly, when faced with a clinical trial report, the astute reader may gain a useful impression of its quality or 'health' by means of an initial broad appraisal before considering any particular aspect in detail. A number of the leading medical journals have defined very strict guidelines on trial report structure, for would-be authors, usually based around the following outline:

- Title
- List of authors, with qualifications and locations
- Trial report summary
- Introduction
- Methods (may include a separate statistics section)
- Results
- Discussion
- Conclusion
- Bibliography
- Other details (source of drugs, acknowledgements, sponsorship and contact point for further information).

The title

This merits careful reading and a few seconds meditation. Good titles have clarity and are intelligible. They are, after all, the keys to the studies which they preface and they should summarize the aims of those studies in as few words as possible. Clear and concise titles often, but not invariably, imply good studies and are usually blessed with the additional virtues of sharpness of definition and relevance. All too often, lured by what appears to be a suitable title in retrieval systems, the hapless reader expends much energy and time to obtain the original article only to find that it is either quite irrelevant or so poor that it is of little use as an information source. It is wise to be wary of 'declaratory' titles, e.g. 'Drug X is effective in the treatment of Y'. This may imply a premature conclusion based on inadequate data. The experienced and competent investigator will avoid this trap. Cryptic titles in which the theme of a study or other article is clouded by obscure terminology, although frequently clever and amusing, can prove an irritating hindrance to retrieval.

The author(s)

One might reasonably expect that authors who are eminent in their field are more likely to impose rigid standards on their clinical research than less experienced and more junior colleagues. How does one assess eminence? Frequency of publication and of citation may suggest an active research involvement while the occupancy of an academic chair and/or a consultancy at a 'centre of excellence' is commonly accepted as a positive indication of reliability. The author has found, particularly as an ethics committee member, that even the most highly respected doctors may become involved in trials that leave much to be desired in terms of design and robustness. Thus it is wise not to use the professional eminence of authors as the sole index of trial quality.

It is worth checking the list of authors, noting the number of contributors and/or any obvious connections with the pharmaceutical industry. The inclusion of a statistician can be the sign of careful planning and may reduce the likelihood of any serious flaws in design or subsequent analysis. A large number of authors from different centres indicates a multi-centre trial, which may merit specially careful appraisal.

The summary

The summary should provide a synopsis of the trial. It should contain information on the aims of the study, preferably defining the hypothesis on which the trial is based. It should also describe the study sample in terms of numbers and disease definition, should summarize the methods which have been used to measure response, provide details of the results and suggest conclusions. An important inclusion is a power statement. This will be discussed later. In the meantime, suffice it to say that the inclusion of a power statement will confirm that attention has been paid to defining a clinically significant response and to recruiting a sufficient number of subjects to demonstrate such a response at chosen levels of chance and probability. It is also important to check the summary for mention of dropouts, i.e. those subjects who, for a variety of reasons, do not complete the trial, and to compare the number of subjects mentioned in the summary with that cited in the main body of the text. Disparities in these and other data may sometimes be found even in the most respected journals.

It is common practice to rely solely on trial report summaries during journal perusal but this is not to be recommended when preparing reviews or dealing with inquiries. Special care needs to be applied when the original is in a foreign language and a bilingual summary is provided. If not prepared by a translator with a good command of English, literal acceptance of the contents of such a summary can prove hazardous.

The introduction

In the introductory section, it is reasonable to expect a brief background to the study in terms of a disease review and the steps in reasoning which prompted the investigators to undertake the study. At this point, it is worth considering whether the trial is designed to answer a clinically relevant issue or is vague in its objectives and is merely being published as part of a paper-chasing career process. Suspicion should be aroused when the tone of the discussion leaps suddenly from the general to the particular with, for example, the abrupt introduction of a particular drug; this might indicate that the trial has a strong promotional bias. The careful reader might also consider undertaking an independent search of relevant literature to exclude the possibility of selective citation, i.e. that the authors have chosen to include references which support their case and to ignore those which do not.

Methods

The methods section is a critical element of the trial report. Defective methodology will seriously impair the quality and hence the reliability of a clinical trial, which no amount of selective argument or statistical manipulation will rectify. In the methods section the authors should amplify the contents of the preceding summary section, by clearly defining such relevant factors as definition of any disease under investigation in the trial, inclusion and exclusion criteria, the number of patients to be recruited, details of treatment and, in particular, the primary and secondary endpoints.

References supporting the choice of methodology can be helpful and if there is any doubt on the part of the reader concerning this aspect of the trial, consultation with a colleague in the relevant speciality may be necessary. The methods of assessment should be clearly described with an emphasis on determination of drug efficacy and of safety. The latter issue can all too easily be relegated to a position of secondary importance. Also it is wise to be wary of an excessive emphasis on statistical analysis since even the most complex analytical techniques cannot rescue a poorly designed study. The definition of a working hypothesis, e.g. that one drug is more effective than another, and a focused investigation to test that hypothesis are the vital elements of clinical investigation and these should be reflected in the contents of the methodology section.

Statistical section

In some clinical trial reports, the section describing the statistical tests that have been used will be included in the methodology section; in others it may receive a separate section. In reading the statistics section, the average reader will recognize some of the simpler tests

Is the trial a multicentre or single site investigation?

In order to recruit sufficient patients for a clinical trial, it may often be necessary to conduct the investigation on a multicentre basis. If this is the case, check that the investigators have recognized and allowed for the various sources of bias that can arise with such a design. These include variations in the precision of clinical assessment between centres, possible variations in laboratory standards and even the effects of location, since diet and climate may play an influential part in disease severity and response to treatment.

Is the study blinded?

Double-blinding, i.e. ensuring that neither the investigator(s) nor the trial subjects are aware which drug is being given to whom (allocation concealment) is an important measure to reduce the possibility of bias (Schulz et al 1995). It is important to check that there are no covert factors in the trial, such as discernible drug side-effects, which might disturb such blinding. When dose frequencies differ between the test drugs, check that this has been compensated for by for example use of a double dummy, i.e. addition of a placebo so that frequencies are the same in both treatment arms.

Is the outcome of the trial positive or negative?

If the outcome of a trial is reported as positive, the grounds for this claim should be evaluated. To claim a difference in effect merely upon an impressive P value, may be unjustified and inspection of the data to determine the magnitude of difference in outcome is advisable. A negative outcome may, similarly, be falsely produced when the trial has insufficient subjects. At this point it is important to stress the important difference between true and false negative studies. The former is one, which because of sound technique and sufficient trial power, allows one to accept the likelihood that there is no difference in effect between two drugs. Note the choice of wording; 'likelihood' is preferable to 'certainty', the latter being a rare commodity in drug trials. A false negative trial produces a negative result because it is too weak to do otherwise. There is evidence that negative studies are less likely to be published than those with positive outcome, a phenomenon aptly known as positive publication bias (Easterbrook et al 1991). This form of bias can introduce serious distortion into treatment assessments and is especially pernicious in the context of meta-analysis.

Are there enough subjects?

The trial report should normally contain a power statement. Based on pilot studies of the likely performance of the test drug, and on the level of response judged to provide a clinically significant advantage, the statistician can calculate the number of subjects who need to be recruited to allow the trial to demonstrate an effect, if one exists. This should, wherever possible, be included as a matter of course.

Are the subjects volunteers or patients?

Data on side-effects or pharmacokinetic profiles obtained from studies on young and healthy volunteers may not be applicable to patients with active disease who may also be advanced in years.

Are inclusion/exclusion criteria defined and are these appropriate?

Subjects are frequently admitted to trials on the basis of certain criteria regarding such variables as age, disease severity or the presence of other diseases including renal and/or hepatic dysfunction. A useful point to consider is whether such criteria render the subjects atypical of those likely to be encountered in routine clinical practice. If this is the case, the trial outcome will be of limited clinical value. The application of excessively rigid exclusion criteria may thus reduce a trial to a mere academic exercise.

Is baseline comparability satisfactory?

Details of the subjects in each arm of a trial should be provided to allow the reader to decide whether there are important differences between the individual groups which might affect outcome. Sometimes the differences may be assessed statistically or, in cases where disparity exists, the effects may be adjusted for by appropriate statistical means. However, such disparity may conceal other differences which, unknown to the investigators and the reader, may also affect response. It is worth perusing baseline comparability tables with great care.

Is the subject description adequate?

Check that adequate information about the trial subjects is provided. Such information should routinely include age, gender, race, disease severity, co-morbidity (presence of other diseases) and concomitant drug treatment.

Have subjects left the trial prematurely?

It is rare to find a trial in which all the subjects who are recruited finish the course. There are many possible reasons why subjects leave a trial but the extent of desertion provides a useful clue as to how the drug is likely to perform in routine clinical use. Although most give up because of unacceptable side-effects, others may leave because they find the drug treatment unpalatable or inconvenient. These are entirely valid reasons for withdrawal and, as with side-effects, have very important clinical implications. Analysis by intention to treat is a common device for dealing with this scenario.

Is the drug dose fixed or variable?

In trials in which the doses of drugs are variable, firm guidelines should be provided for dose determination since such variation may obviously affect subject response.

Are the doses of drugs comparable?

The doses of drugs used in trials should be checked to exclude the possibility that they have been taken from extreme ends of their respective normal dose ranges, a distortion which could introduce a serious bias in trial outcome.

Are the treatments distinguishable?

The investigators should provide an assurance that the various treatments under evaluation are not readily distinguishable by means of taste, colour, appearance or side-effects, thus preserving trial blindness.

Are sufficient drug details provided?

Merely to provide details of drug dosage is insufficient. The reader should be told the source of supply, details of any special formulation, the route of administration and frequency. Such detail is essential if the results of drug trials are to be used to support the launch of a new drug, a situation in which it is vital that the test drug and the marketed presentation are comparable.

Is the comparator appropriate?

In assessing the efficacy of a new drug, comparison needs to be made with another drug, treatment or placebo. Volumes have been written concerning the role of the placebo in clinical trials. Sometimes it is described as an 'inactive' treatment. This is often proved incorrect, since in certain diseases, irritable bowel being a good example, the placebo response can prove considerable. Generally, the trial comparator should be a treatment which is recognized as effective and is routinely used. A placebo comparator should normally be reserved for situations in which no other treatment is available or where therapeutic activity alone needs to be demonstrated, as during preparation for licensing applications.

Who measures the response?

Several investigators may be involved in assessing patient response. In such a case, some evidence of reproducibility of assessment technique is desirable but is often wanting. When patients make their own assessments, for example by use of symptom diaries, it is wise to suspect a considerable measure of variation unless such records can be validated.

Are assessments numerical or descriptive?

Many important measures of response in clinical trials are descriptive rather than numerical. Depression, for example, is hard to quantify and resort is normally made to recognized scales which attempt to describe the severity of this illness in a defined manner. Similarly, analogue scales may be used to assess pain. A problem can arise, however, when crude methods of symptom assessment, such as 'mild', 'moderate' or 'severe' are used to derive numerical values, which can convey a spurious impression of precision. Ensure that you are happy with the precision and relevance of the measures described in a trial report.

Are percentages reported?

Although percentages are commonly used in reporting results, these can be used as a smokescreen for small values. Never accept a percentage value without checking the original numerical values on which the percentage is based.

Is the trial randomized?

Most clinical trial reports will mention randomization; far fewer may describe the method used. This is an essential part of the trial report and its absence may reasonably leave one to assume that an inappropriate method may have been employed, such as allocation by birth date. The validity of the statistical tests used to analyse the trial data depend on random allocation of treatments so that selection bias is excluded. Simple randomization, by use of tables or computer-based programmes may not ensure that treatments within a trial are evenly allocated, leading to an imbalance in the number of subjects within each treatment arm. The use of block randomization provides a means of achieving comparable numbers in the different arms of a trial; stratified randomization can be used when a subgroup hypothesis is to be tested by randomizing separately within each subgroup of the trial (Roberts & Torgerson 1998).

Is there evidence of bias?

Bias, in the context of the clinical trial, is any influence that distorts the performance or interpretation of that trial possibly leading to an incorrect conclusion. Several potential sources of bias in relation to choice of subjects and drug dosage have already been mentioned in earlier parts of this chapter. Bias may be deliberate or inadvertent, the latter including both accidental bias and unrecognized personal bias.

During teaching sessions on bias in trials, the author frequently uses the analogy of life drawing and painting. Those who pursue this branch of art will know that the nude is extremely difficult to draw or paint. The complex structural relationships of the human form demand care in observation to achieve success. The task becomes even more difficult when the model is sitting or lying down, since this introduces the problem of 'foreshortening' as the accepted size relationships of limbs and torso are distorted. The experienced artist will preface an approach to the easel with a prolonged study of the model, thus avoiding the errors that first impressions can convey. A further important point is that there is no standard human shape. The artist must adjust to the individual characteristics of the model. Last but not least, budding life artists must learn to depict what they see, not what they know. A lifetime of familiarity with the appearance of the human form, albeit normally clothed, interferes with the process of accurate artistic depiction and demands the development of skill in detached observation.

Clearly, there are lessons here for trial investigators. The task of designing and conducting a clinical trial is, like that of the life artist, a profoundly complex process with many pitfalls. Even to miss one apparently small anomaly can spell disaster. In assessing the response of patients in a trial, and in analysing the results of such assessment, our interpretation will be influenced by our own personal mental filter, which will preferentially select those aspects of the emergent data that match our preconceptions and personal bias (hence the spirited arguments in the correspondence columns of journals). Familiarity with a particular area of medicine can hinder rather than assist the performance of a sufficiently robust and impartial trial. The investigators are too close to the subject to see it in a dispassionate manner. Results that do not match our expectations (rather like the foreshortening of our life model) may be 'corrected' by, for example, excluding values that are outside the normal expected range, or by avoidance of publication. Like the model, patients are individuals with their own drug response characteristics.

There are many sources of bias in clinical trials (Sackett 1979) some of which may be entirely missed by the relevant investigators. It may happen that they have sampled from a population of subjects with some characteristic which will cause an atypical drug reaction (possibly a genetic feature linked to ethnicity). Choice of an inappropriate comparator may bias the results in favour of the test drug. To compare the effects of a non-steroidal anti-inflammatory drug with a simple analgesic in the relief of arthritic stiffness would be an example. Studies of disease associations, if confined to samples of hospital patients, may suffer from Berkson's Bias or Berkson's Fallacy (Berkson 1946), which relates to different inherent rates of hospital admission for individual diseases. An empirical demonstration of this source of bias has been published; although possibly somewhat esoteric, it does have implications in the field of adverse drug reactions (Roberts et al 1978).

Finally, it is important to stress that bias is not confined to promotional pharmaceutical material. One commonly reads that a particular source of information is 'unbiased' when what is meant is that there is no commercial influence. This does not exclude the possibility of distortion resulting from the personal bias of its authors. Covert commercial bias in publication has been the subject of a number of articles and comments (Smith 1994, Smith 1998).

Statistics

It is very noticeable that the statistical aspects of a clinical trial report or proposed investigation are rarely touched on by most members of ethics or drug and therapeutics committees, especially when a statistician is present. This is understandable. For most of us, the science of statistics is seen as a complex and obscure subject, characterized by its own curious terminology and weighed down by voluminous equations. Statisticians have their own distinct and largely unintelligible language, which often hinders their communication with other professions. While statistics is an absorbing and even stimulating area of mathematical science, its appeal may be limited and for many drug information specialists an extensive study of this science would be an indulgence in time which they can ill afford.

With the average reader in mind, the following brief section is biased towards principles rather than formulae and is presented with the hope that it may urge the reader to further study.

In preparing any clinical trial, thought must be given to the population of potential trial subjects from whom a sample will be drawn. The target population will be defined in terms of those factors (e.g. type of disease and its severity) considered relevant to the proposed study. Much will hinge on the quality of the sample, which will depend on many factors. The more subjects whom we include in our sample the more likely it is that we reduce the disturbing effects of differences between individuals and the more likely it is that the mean values for treatment response will be representative of the population from which our sample is drawn.

For many types of data, the statistician can test the reliability of a mean by calculation of the standard error of the mean, which is calculated from the sample size and scatter of values within the sample. By adding and subtracting approximately two (1.96 to be precise) standard errors of the mean to and from the mean response value, we obtain a very useful statistic which we call the 95% confidence interval. We can be 95% certain that the 'true' mean of the population from which our sample is derived lies within the limits defined by the confidence intervals (and we are also 5% certain that it lies outside those limits!). If we have a good sample, which is reasonably large and within which there are not too extreme values, our confidence intervals will be narrow and our mean value can be accepted with a reasonable measure of confidence. If we have too few subjects, with widely scattered responses, our confidence intervals will be wide and we will be less happy about the reliability of our mean value. We would conclude that our trial is weak and susceptible to a type II error in failing to distinguish between the effects of two treatments even when a difference in effect exists. If we were sufficiently misguided to attempt numerous repeated analyses of our data with various statistical tests until we found one which produced a significant outcome, our results would be afflicted with a type I error, i.e. a positive outcome when one does not exist.

In most trials, results will be qualified by reference to a P value as a measure of clinical significance. Increasingly this is reported as a number rather than the traditional 'less than' estimate. The P value gives the probability that we have observed our results when the null hypothesis (that there is no difference in effects between treatments being compared in the trial) is true. Thus a P value of 0.01 tells us that there is a 1/100 chance that our trial results will indicate a difference in drug effect even when such a difference does not exist. The significance of our result thus conveys an estimate of the reliability that can be placed on our result, but this does not necessarily confirm that it is a real effect or even further, that it is *clinically* significant.

The type of statistical test which we use is influenced by many considerations including the normality or otherwise of our data. Distribution curves, obtained by plotting the number of individuals with a given value (ordinate) against the individual values (abscissa) for normal data show a curve which is approximately bell-shaped. Such data show normal (or Gaussian) distribution. For such data, use of a parametric test will be appropriate. Marked distortion of our curve to the left or right (skewing) indicates that our data are more appropriately analysed using non-parametric tests unless we normalize them (e.g. by log transformation). Where data are skewed, use of the median (the value that lies in the middle when individual values are arranged in ascending order) may be a more meaningful measure of centrality (i.e. a more representative sample value) than the mean which can be heavily influenced by extreme values (outliers). Over recent years, there has been a move away from sole reliance on P values to a greater emphasis on confidence intervals. These are much more informative about the quality of data.

As you read more trial reports, you will find instances where apparently similar investigations have yielded contradictory results. Recognition of the fact that reliance on the result of a single trial can be misleading has led to increasing use of meta-analysis which involves the pooling of data from a number of small trials and analyses to obtain a new estimate of effect. Such analyses have to be conducted within firm guidelines to be reliable. A number of instances have occurred where the results of such analyses have been contradicted by subsequent large-scale trials (megatrials). Where this has occurred, various explanations have been offered such as differences between patients and dosing schedules but it has also been recognized that positive publication bias, mentioned earlier in this chapter, can have a disastrous effect. Remember that erroneous meta-analyses are not merely an academic curiosity. The results of such analyses if applied to patient care can have dangerous consequences. The results of meta-analyses are commonly presented as odds ratios which describe the proportional response to various treatments. These too, can be qualified by confidence intervals to provide some assessment of reliability. Finally, care is needed in dealing with measures such as absolute risk reduction, relative risk reduction and NNT (number needed to treat) which although simple in concept, can cause endless confusion.

Promotional information

In this section there is repetition of several points of assessment that were made in the sections on clinical trials. The distinction between promotional literature and the contents of even the most eminent medical journals can be blurred. Clinical trial reports may be subject to some measure of commercial influence and even seemingly dispassionate reviews of drug treatment have occasionally been criticized on the grounds of commercial bias.

In matching an evaluation of clinical trials of a new drug with the promotion of that drug, it is very useful to obtain a copy of current promotional brochures, since these are likely to contain the key messages which are being used to promote the drug. These can then be checked against the original trial reports for accuracy.

It is wise to be very wary of references included in promotional material. Those listed as 'data on file' or 'to be published' should prompt a request for further information. A predominance of old references may indicate that the drug has been 'sitting on the shelf' for a long period. Drug promotions, which are supported by material in abstract form, may be very difficult to evaluate since the abstract is unlikely to contain sufficient detail to enable a judgement of worth to be made. Furthermore, a reference list composed mainly of obscure and inaccessible journal titles may be a reasonable cause for suspicion.

Marketing is a very sophisticated art and nowhere is this seen more effectively than in the advertisements common to most medical journals. Psychological skills are used in conjunction with the minimum of text to impress potential prescribers. Important details of dosage, adverse effects and precautions are included but often in small print. The graphics used in drug advertisements are frequently compelling and even seductive. Sometimes promotional literature takes the form of interactive material such as a face which alters its expression as the brochure is opened, eyes which move or 'pop-up' illustrations. The numerous memorabilia (pens, paper weights, scribbling pads etc.) bearing the name of a particular drug are a further well-established means of brand image reinforcement.

When reading promotional brochures or during discussion with drug representatives, it is important to seek out the key points of distinction claimed for the drug and to request evidence to support such claims. This should be rigorously evaluated and any points of concern discussed with the relevant medical department. Pharmaceutical representatives can be an invaluable source of information and may actually welcome exchange with a questioning and interactive professional. However, a detailed study in the USA concluded that statements made by pharmaceutical representatives are not always accurate (Ziegler et al 1995). As with all other sources of information, a politely critical approach is recommended.

In the UK, the ABPI Code of Practice provides helpful guidance on assessing promotional drug claims and the reports of the Prescription Medicines Code of Practice Authority make

Lastly, we need to develop a strategic plan for the future and decide to whom the services need to be promoted, including both existing and potential valuable customers.

Using two case histories, we can see example models for both the pharmaceutical industry and healthcare services. These case histories were developed by Andrew Robson for the first intake of students for the Diploma in Pharmaceutical Information Management at City University London, UK, 1997. By looking at these, and by considering the points given above, you can begin to develop your own effective business case.

Justifying a pharmaceutical industry information service

Imagine that you manage a pharmaceutical industry information service and that a proposal has been made to outsource this service. What arguments would you put forward to retain the service in-house? We can use this scenario to begin to develop a business case. We would first need measures of success and productivity. Third-party endorsement of the existing services would also be important. It would be desirable to consider ways in which the service could be improved. It would also be essential to consider, as fairly as possible, the likely consequences of outsourcing the service.

Unique Selling Points include:

- searching skills of in-house staff
- cost effectiveness of the service
- offering a proactive service
- flexibility of response from knowledge of the company business
- breadth and depth of product knowledge only possible within the company
- detailed knowledge of the company business, including confidential information and company culture
- sensitivity to company politics
- current awareness expertise
- good interpersonal skills of staff providing the service.

Reasons not to outsource include:

- cost of outsourcing the service
- confidentiality of information, including knowledge of R&D products pre-launch.
- gaining and maintaining trust from external staff party to confidential information
- possible conflicts of interest in positioning information
- some services could not be outsourced, e.g. approval of promotional material
- loss of knowledge about customer base and issues arising
- loss of close contact with customers
- loss of knowledge base within the company, including current awareness
- loss of flexibility by being tied to fixed contracts
- need for new job functions to implement, control and audit contracted services
- loss of rapid response ability.

Advantages of retaining an internal service include:

- retain a central point of contact
- retain a central feedback source
- retain a route of gaining excellent staff who have a wide range of skills and qualifications that can be of use elsewhere within the organization as a career development path.

Measurements needed to support the business case include:

- statistics on basic services offered (e.g. number of enquiries, training sessions, customer base etc.)
- customer surveys

- monitor number of questions and repeat customers to show customer need and endorsement.

Competitor analysis

Potential competitors might include:

- external services (e.g. literature alerts from suppliers, helplines offered by patient associations or drug information units, commercial call centres)
- internal services (e.g. corporate information groups, non-use by key customers, informal networks).

There is a need to assess competitor skills and costs, and to research their strengths and weaknesses.

Strategic plan

- Decide upon preferred option.
- Promote value of services to senior management team.
- Support proposal with hard data.
- Provide regular briefings (written or oral) on service, its commercial value and business outcomes (e.g. customer satisfaction).
- Keep up to date with the competition (e.g. external outsourcing opportunities, call centres etc.).

Justification of a drug information service in a hospital

A group of Diploma in Pharmaceutical Information Management students was asked to justify a hospital drug information service. This is the case that they created.

Customer base

The customer base can be determined from an enquiry database and would include:

- hospital doctors, pharmacists and nurses
- general practitioners
- retail pharmacists
- health authority staff, e.g. pharmaceutical and medical advisors.

USPs within the hospital environment include:

- objective evaluation of information
- proactive service
- excellent communication skills
- practical pharmacy and clinical experience
- local knowledge of health services
- familiarity with IT systems to support the organization
- knowledge of a range of information sources and skills to use them efficiently
- access to the national drug information pharmacists' network.

Benefits of providing a hospital drug information service include:

- improving patient care and risk management (e.g. using drug safety information)
- financial considerations—involvement in formulary decisions leads to more rational prescribing and effective use of healthcare resources
- use of information reduces patient disease complications
- improved patient care (hard to measure).

Competitors

Competitors could include clinical pharmacists. Despite their specific skills and competencies, they may not have the knowledge of all the information sources and training of drug information pharmacists.

Other competitors include pharmaceutical industry information professionals. However, they lack local knowledge, may have a narrow focus of knowledge on their own products and may be considered to have bias towards their own products.

A business case will require an analysis of comparative competitor strengths and weaknesses. This will help predict the threat that they pose and what opportunities can be exploited.

Possible future directions

- Developing new customers including health authority advisors, directors of public health etc.
- Use of IT for business advantage and to train others.
- Promotion of services to end users so they answer their own questions.
- Targeting services towards the top team within the hospital.
- Develop clarity of role within the department and outside.
- Gain more customer feedback.
- Be more proactive in services.

By using this structured approach to justification of services, a suitable business case can be put forward and the staffing levels adjusted according to executive approval.

Recruitment

Recruitment of high quality staff is a key responsibility of any information manager. Choosing the right person is vital to building and developing a successful team, thereby ensuring that the services provided are of the required quality.

Recruitment alternatives

The process starts by determining what resource is required. It could be that a staff member has left the company or has been promoted and has to be replaced. Alternatively, extra staff may be needed to cover new research areas, product launches or line extensions. The first question that a manager needs to ask is whether a new member of staff is really needed. Does the department carry out any unnecessary tasks or responsibilities? Could the work be delegated or outsourced? If so, these unnecessary responsibilities can be eliminated, after proper consideration, and the released resource can be used to cover the new additional activities.

Once it has been determined that extra or replacement staff are necessary, and assuming that recruitment has been justified by the manager and approved by higher management, then consideration needs to be given to the type of staff needed. Do they need to be full-time permanent members? If the work is of short duration (e.g. maternity cover, product launch, line extension), then contract staff may be more appropriate.

Alternative arrangements to permanent staff include:

- contract staff via an agency
- secretarial temporary staff
- secondments from within the company (e.g. sales representatives, research scientists etc.)
- students—holiday or sandwich students
- outsourcing
- part-time staff or job share arrangements.

Selection of staff is a major responsibility for any manager and must be done well to ensure future success. There are many books and training programmes that will provide managers with the skills and competencies for recruitment. Some suggested books include Buzan (1995), Fleming (1997) and Russell-Jones (1995). Whilst this chapter cannot hope to train managers in these skills, the main points will be discussed.

Recruitment process

Job specification

Recruitment of staff is a six-stage process (see Fig. 7.1). The initial stage is to prepare a job specification. This should detail the job purpose and the appropriate skills, previous experience, qualifications and competencies of the person being sought. Other critical factors need to be included. Examples might include need to travel, a clean driving licence, etc. Personality, outlook and values should also be considered.

This stage can be overlooked and yet it is vital if the process is to be successful. The job specification is used to choose interview candidates and decide final selection. If there are any complaints about the selection process by a potential candidate (e.g. age, racial, disability or sex discrimination), then the job specification will be needed in conjunction with all the candidates' details to show that selection was objective rather than subjective. The job specification will also be useful in preparing an advertisement.

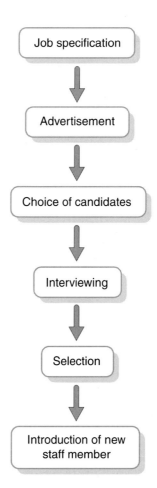

Figure 7.1
Recruitment process

Chapter 19 covers the skills and competencies of information personnel and can be used as a guide in preparing a job specification. Companies may have a specific format that is used. It is also necessary to consider and clarify what are the salary range and benefits packages that go with the job. The personnel or human resources (HR) department can also help with this process.

Advertisement

Having set the job specification, the next step is to consider how you will manage the recruitment and advertising process. New posts may need to be advertised within the company first to make best use of company resources and to tap into the pool of talent within the company. Word of mouth is another route to take—you or your staff may know of someone. If these routes are not successful, then external advertisement is the next step.

Various recruitment agencies specialize in pharmaceutical industry or information professional appointments. There are several advantages in using an agency. It will do most of the recruitment on the customer's behalf including advertising (and help with composing the advertisement), initial screening of the applicants against the defined job specification, initial professional interviewing and will advise on candidate selection. This can be an advantage in the absence of support within the company (e.g. HR support) or if the manager has insufficient time or recruitment experience. Balanced against this is the cost, which is usually dependent upon successful recruitment.

Alternatively, the decision can be made to manage the process within the company, usually with the support and guidance of the HR department. Composition of a recruitment advertisement is the next step. The job specification will help define the key information to get across but this is an opportunity to sell the job, department and company and so a different style of writing is required. HR departments may have an agency that helps with copywriting and design. The advertisement should specify a (realistic) closing date for applications. It should also give a contact point from which applicants can obtain further information (e.g. company website).

Pharmaceutical information advertisements in the UK are usually placed in a number of journals. The main journals or newsletters include *New Scientist*, *Pharmaceutical Journal* and *AIOPI News*. Increasingly, jobs can also be posted on the internet (e.g. InPharm, Pharmiweb). Consideration should be made of cost and the audience that you want to reach. Administrative or secretarial jobs may be advertised in the local press.

Candidate choice

Assuming that the advertisement yields a number of candidates who are interested in the post, choice of interview candidates is the next step. Each curriculum vitae (résumé) must be checked against the job specification. It is easy to be influenced by a well-presented CV. It is worth looking for discrepancies and gaps. What information seems to be missing? What has been misrepresented? A significant proportion of people will overemphasize or fabricate achievements or claim others' achievements for themselves.

It is often easier to weed out completely unsuitable candidates first which will then leave potentials for interview. It is essential that candidates are not discriminated against on the basis of age, sex, race or disability. It is useful to briefly annotate CVs to explain why applicants were not selected in case there is any follow-up.

There is no ideal number of people to interview—it may be that there are only two lead candidates, in which case both should be seen. If there are more than six suitable candidates, a further selection procedure is necessary to reduce the number. For example, if the work requires very good telephone skills and rapport, then it might be suitable to arrange a telephone interview, giving the candidates sufficient notice to prepare themselves. Once the final short list is produced, it is time to arrange the interviews.

Interviewing

Interviewing potential staff face to face is still the main process for selecting staff, despite the fact that there is an element of subjective selection rather than objective choice. First impressions can influence decisions. Therefore it is important to try to overcome this tendency and to use as objective a process as possible. Many management books cover this topic extensively (e.g. McBride & Clark, 1996), providing further insight and, in some cases, exercises. Assessment centres are also used, but rarely for recruitment of information staff.

Sitting on the interviewer's side of the desk is still strange and definitely nerve-wracking for many managers! Here are some useful tips to get started.

The first point to consider is setting—where will the interview be conducted? Ideally it needs to be in a room with no interruptions (people or telephones). Refreshments will help to create a welcoming atmosphere. As you may both be nervous, a drink will also help deal with dry mouth. Consider placement of tables or desks, chairs, lighting etc. If you really want to relax someone, you may wish to remove the physical barrier of a desk.

Preparation is always necessary. Use the job specification to prepare some essential questions on areas that it is important to cover, e.g. previous experience, achievements, feedback from current manager etc. For each individual, it is important to read through the CV, looking for areas that you do not understand or wish to explore further. Do the dates of jobs/degrees make sense? Are there any gaps and why? Are there any questions about the achievements in various positions etc? Questions must be relevant and not stem from prejudice.

It is a good idea to start the interview by general social chatter about the person's journey or some other neutral questions. The aim is to relax the candidate as much as possible and get him/her into the swing of answering questions. It is useful to start by outlining the programme and timings for the session, especially if it may take more than a few hours. Ideally details would have been outlined in the letter of invitation to the interview.

Initial questions on education are a good start—asking the candidate to summarize his or her education can provide an indication of ability to précis information orally. Next, move on to employment history to focus on previous and current duties and responsibilities, achievements, career development, feedback received etc. Other areas to probe include motivation and aspirations, leisure activities (does this person prefer team activities, leadership roles, solitary hobbies or sports?) and availability.

Judicious use of open and closed questions will help. Open questions will probe areas in depth (e.g. Why did you chose to work for XYZ company? What do you enjoy about your current position? Describe the difficulties you have experienced in your previous post). Closed questions will help confirm facts and ensure brief replies.

Silence is a useful way to encourage someone to open up further should you wish more depth to an answer. Body language is a powerful tool in interviewing. Use of smiles to relax interviewees, nods to indicate understanding, etc. will improve the success of the interview. Body language is a fascinating topic and as space does not allow further detail, it is worth consulting books on the topic (e.g. Pease 1997).

It is worth taking some notes during the interview and summarizing your findings. If you have to interview many candidates, differentiating between them may become a problem unless you have some notes upon which you will base a decision. They may also be useful for providing specific feedback to candidates who ask why they were unsuccessful.

The interview structure may include time to meet other staff members and to be interviewed by them, if relevant. It is useful to gain other people's impressions and to provide an opportunity for candidates to meet their potential future colleagues. There may also be the opportunity to conduct some situational tests, though they may be relevant only at second interview stage as they take time. For example, if the job specification requires writing skills, you may wish to ask candidates to write a short piece. When assessing such work you should make allowance for the fact that they were performing under pressure.

Close the interview by inviting the candidate to ask questions and outlining the next stages, with timings. For example, the successful candidate will be contacted in two weeks time when you have completed the first round of interviews. Keep to arranged timings. Also be prepared to give all candidates feedback on why they were unsuccessful.

Selection

To select the best candidate, it is essential to match people against the job specification. If there are two people who are equally matched, deciding which are the most important criteria will help separate the candidates. If the right person has not been found, managers should not be tempted to recruit a poor candidate or they will regret the choice in time to come. There are alternatives that may be put in place whilst the recruitment strategy or tactics are changed. Use of contract staff is one example.

Introduction of new staff

Think very carefully how you will introduce the new member of staff into the team and plan initial training. This will set the pattern for this person's employment with you. It is important to get off to a good start.

Staff development

Every member of staff within the team should have a development plan, regardless of level or experience. Self-actualization is a very powerful motivator and will help retain staff within a team. Whilst staff continue to be developed and learn new skills, they will prefer to stay with a company or team. So how do managers develop their staff? While this is discussed from an individual standpoint in Chapter 19, the slant in this chapter is to consider the role of the manager.

Sadly, not all managers believe in the importance of staff development. They may think that they have insufficient time or may not know how to develop others. Some managers may think that they will lose staff to another organization once they are fully trained. In some cases, they may not want their staff to be better skilled than themselves. Excuses of insufficient budget for training courses are inadequate. Staff development is not just about attending training courses but can be implemented using imaginative methods.

Alternatively, managers may find situations where a staff member may take no interest in developing his or her skills and will not attend appropriate training courses. In situations like these, it is necessary to be pragmatic and realize that you cannot force people and it would be counterproductive to do so. Staff need to be made aware of the consequences of their actions. The team member may not acquire the skills suitable for promotion or there may be an issue about basic job capability. It is worth recognizing that the most successful teams are those with a suitable mixture of capabilities, personalities and experience levels. Not everyone in the team needs to be a rising star!

So how do managers develop their staff? To start, they have to determine the areas of development. These should naturally fall out from the process of objective setting and assessment against objectives. If there is a mismatch, i.e. performance is less than that required, then a development need has been identified. Identification of development needs can also come from career aspirations. If someone has been doing an information job for a year or two, it is probably time to prepare for the next step in development, taking into consideration ability and potential. The development objectives and plan must be agreed between both parties, manager and team member.

Having identified areas for development, the next step is to choose an appropriate method. This is covered in Chapter 19 on career development. To summarize, methods may include:

- mentoring
- coaching by manager or peer
- role plays
- reading
- videos
- manuals or standard operating procedures
- being 'thrown in the deep end', with support
- shadowing
- deputizing
- talking to experts
- making mistakes
- committee/task force work
- training courses.

Not every method will suit every person. One of the skills of management is knowing how people learn and which method to use with different staff at different times. Space does not permit this topic to be covered in the detail that would do it justice. The management books listed at the end of this chapter provide further information. Situational leadership skills are very relevant to this topic (see Blanchard et al 1985).

Budget management

Managers are judged on many performance measures and one key area is usually budget management. For example, you may be required to bring in your budget at year-end without overshooting or undershooting by more than 5% of the total.

It may be a topic that initially worries a newly appointed manager because of lack of experience. However, armed with knowledge of a few financial principles and a commitment to managing the process well, any manager can successfully manage a budget.

There will be aspects of budget management that will be specific for the company. These include the dates of the financial year and planning cycles, budgetary systems, principle of cross charging of services or certain costs etc.

Let us explore the topic by imagining that you are a newly recruited information manager. What do you need to know?

Planning cycle for following year

Where are you in the cycle? Has the budget for the following year already been set or is this process to come? It is useful to know the dates so that you can plan ahead accordingly. To prepare for the following year(s), you need to know current spending trends and environmental factors that could influence the budget (e.g. size of product portfolio, product launches, new customers or services, downsizing etc). There is often an accountant in the finance department who can provide guidance in the process but only you will know the factors influencing your budget.

Budget structure

What is the total budget and how is it broken down? Many companies use specific cost codes to assign costs to particular functions, e.g. staff training, travel, hotel accommodation, online searching bills, journal costs, etc. It is important to use the correct code for specific purchases so that accurate spending costs can be tracked, rather than looking at which cost codes have money within them and therefore can be raided! This will help in the process of setting budgets for years to come and it will ensure that costs are accurately reflected.

Cross-charges

Some costs from the information department may be charged to other departments or functions (often called cost centres) if those other functions are entirely responsible for the costs. Examples might include journal or book purchases, conference costs etc. Whether this is done depends upon company philosophy. If the information department does cross-charge its costs elsewhere, it may well in turn be cross-charged for costs it incurs. To justify cross-charges, specific information needs to be collected. For example, if journal subscription costs are cross-charged to other departments or divisions, the information centre will need to collect accurate measures of journal use to be able to apportion costs. The effort involved needs to be carefully considered. Collecting and analysing such data is time-consuming and it is not the primary purpose of an information department.

Unplanned expenditure

Despite the best of intentions, there may be situations where unexpected costs are incurred. Examples might be replacement of staff on long-term absence, equipment failure, need for a new service or expensive journal. In these situations it is best to work closely with a contact point in finance as well as your own manager so that they are alerted to and can agree the additional expenditure. In certain circumstances, the annual budget may be adjusted upwards to include the new expenditure.

Phasing of purchase

For an information centre, many of the costs may be fixed for each month. On a monthly basis, expenditure on salaries and benefits, online costs, travel etc. will be fairly steady. However, there will also be annual costs (e.g. annual invoice for journal subscriptions, database maintenance fee etc.) and irregular costs (e.g. conference fees, project costs, training costs etc.). Again, it is important to alert the finance department to the phasing of costs as they may wish to spread them throughout the year (e.g. journal subscriptions) for costly items.

The basics of managing a budget are roughly similar to managing your own personal finances. There is fixed income (the budget), against which costs are deducted. Monthly statements are often available to track costs and budget performance. By checking the performance of the budget, further planning may be necessary. Do you have sufficient budget to fund purchases later in the year?

If there is an excess of budget (i.e. unspent), the finance department may wish to reclaim it to fund other departments and costs centres.

Teams

It takes a team to make a dream. (Sign outside NASA Mission Control, Texas.)

The need for effective teams and teamworking has never been greater in both the pharmaceutical industry and healthcare systems. This is due to the development of complex situations and issues, increased customer expectations, role uncertainty and competitive pressures.

Any information manager needs to know how to build and get the best from teams. But what is a team? How does it differ from a group? Teams or groups are both collections of people who have a common purpose (or set of individual tasks) which tends to be explicit (see Adair, 1987). A team tends to cooperate in such a way that synergy arises and achieves more than the sum total of the individual contributions. Teams tend to be more flexible than larger groups, take more risks and explore new areas. Teams generate a wider range of ideas than individuals alone. They help each other develop their skills and gain confidence

(Fleming 1996). As groups do not have the same behaviour within them, they do not enjoy the same level of success.

Managers need to know about the two key stages of team life cycles: teambuilding and teamworking. First they need to know how to build a team. This involves giving people a sense of purpose, helping them to get to know each other, recognizing skills and abilities as well as establishing a method of working (Fleming 1996). Once the team has been built, teamworking is the next phase and it involves staff cooperating, sharing ideas, being open and supporting each other.

Teambuilding

Teambuilding is used to create new teams or to review the performance of existing teams. Teams are needed when people need to work closely together on real tasks, when there is a problem which needs to be resolved and the solution is not clear or when there is rapid change.

Recruitment into the team is one key stage. Not every team leader will have a choice of team members. This sets a challenge for the leader and will test his/her leadership skills to ensure that the team works effectively.

It is important that the team is of the optimum size according to the function. Groups above 15 members become ineffective (see Fleming, 1996). It is also important that the members are not too similar in their styles of behaviour, specialist knowledge or functions. Successful teams have members with different roles and responsibilities. Time should be taken to analyse who best fits particular roles to ensure peak performance. It is essential to have the right person doing the right job.

This philosophy has been widely explored in management theory and practice. There are many psychological models and psychometric tests available to profile people and their natural styles, which can help in group or team analysis.

Two tests used widely include Belbin's team styles (Belbin, 1996) and the Myers Briggs Type Indicator. Both can be useful in particular situations when forming teams or analysing the team members' styles. It is important that trained personnel (e.g. human resources or training departments) carry out psychometric tests to avoid incorrect or unprofessional individual feedback. Belbin's team styles (see Table 7.1) will give some information about the individual's preferred ways of working within a team. Taking together all the Belbin scores, it is useful to identify overall team strengths and weakness. For example an analysis of a

Table 7.1 *Belbin's team styles*

Role	
Chairman	Controls the way the team moves towards its objectives and makes best use of team resources
Company Worker	Turns concepts and plans into practical procedures. Carries out agreed plans systematically and efficiently
Completer–Finisher	Maintains sense of urgency, searches for work requiring attention and makes sure the team does not take on unagreed extra work nor misses important tasks
Monitor–Evaluator	Analyses problems, evaluates ideas and suggestions to ensure team makes balanced decisions
Plant	Suggests new ideas and strategies, concentrating on major issues
Resource Investigator	Explores and reports on ideas, developments and resources outside the group
Shaper	Shapes the way in which the team effort is applied. Directs attention to the setting of priorities and objectives
Teamworker	Supports others in their strengths, improves communications and fosters team spirit

Adapted from information in Belbin 1996

team using Belbin's test could identify that the team is missing someone who ensures that tasks are completed. This could be the trigger for certain members to fulfil this role. Not everyone is enamoured of these models, however. Adair (1987) cautions against too much reliance on these tests in team situations.

Once the team is assembled, it is time to start building them into a cohesive force. First the team objectives must be set. The team needs to know:

- the task(s) that need to be completed (what)
- completion time (when)
- purpose (why) and environment in which the work needs to be completed
- objective(s) must be clear, specific, challenging and measurable
- what resources are available?
- what will success look like?

Within pharmaceutical information management, specific objectives could be a project (e.g. develop a current awareness service, re-engineer a business process etc.) or a daily task (e.g. provide an information enquiry service for research customers).

It is crucial to involve all team members to ensure a successful outcome. To do this, the manager must learn about the skills, competencies and experience of every member of the team. Together, it is important to create a vision of the objective, ideally using as many senses as possible, e.g. pictures and diagrams, written material and discussions. Different people are influenced by different senses (e.g. sight, hearing etc.) and this method can increase the chance of successful uptake of information and personal involvement.

It is important that team members are set clear roles and responsibilities to avoid unnecessary duplication of effort as well as ensuring that all tasks are adequately covered. They need to know how they fit together to form a whole team, rather like an orchestra.

As well as determining the objective (the 'what'), the team also needs to decide on how they will work together (the 'how' or process). They can learn from past experience of what has been successful as well as unsuccessful. Factors favouring success include:

- work processes should be as straightforward as possible
- team members should be flexible and open in their behaviour
- work should not be overplanned
- standards of performance should be agreed.

Review of progress against targets is a critical stage and can boost performance if used effectively. Successful teams review processes and look at ways to do more, faster, better. Importantly, successful teams also celebrate achievements and successes along the way and have fun!

Leaders and managers

Already we have started to define ways in which teams work effectively. However there is not always a smooth transition from a new team to high performance and outstanding achievements. The role of the leader is critical.

How do managers and leaders differ? Various management gurus have expanded upon the difference at length. Managers manage resources whereas leaders help groups to achieve their common tasks, they maintain the team as a unified group and ensure that each individual contributes his/her best (Adair 1987).

Leaders challenge people, whilst ensuring that appropriate support is available. Strong team members can help those who have weaknesses. Leaders rotate jobs and responsibilities to extend skills and competencies. They create opportunities for others. They lead from the front, knowing what needs to be done and inspiring others to do it and to extend their possibilities and performance.

They know how to listen, act appropriately, explain things and they know when to withdraw. They know how to motivate others and delegate appropriately.

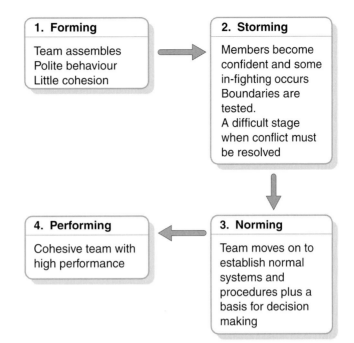

1. Forming

Team assembles
Polite behaviour
Little cohesion

2. Storming

Members become
confident and some
in-fighting occurs
Boundaries are
tested.
A difficult stage
when conflict must
be resolved

4. Performing

Cohesive team with
high performance

3. Norming

Team moves on to
establish normal
systems and
procedures plus a
basis for decision
making

Figure 7.2 *Model of team behaviour in transition*

Leaders also need to be followers. They need to learn and extend their own skills. With a fast pace of change, they must learn rapidly, seeking out development opportunities and experience. Leaders need to be open to challenge and be challenged. Asking the question 'why?' can encourage rethinking. Leaders ask for personal feedback.

Leaders need to understand about group behaviour and influencing styles and they should use different behaviours according to the situation (see Blanchard et al 1985 for further details about situational leadership).

Use of effective leadership styles will enable a team to progress from teambuilding to teamworking.

Teamworking

A useful model of team behaviour in transition is the forming—storming—norming—performing pattern. This is shown in Figure 7.2.

The behaviour of the leader will need to vary according to the stage. For example, during the vital storming stage, the leader needs to know how to successfully resolve conflict. Focusing upon the work to be done can help defuse some situations as long as fundamental differences are not ignored. A certain amount of conflict is healthy to generate new ideas and to challenge existing work practices. However, it becomes unhealthy if bullying, time wasting or losing sight of the main tasks occurs.

The leader can help move teams more rapidly through these transition phases and thus promote teamworking. Not all teams will progress beyond the storming phase!

Service development

Service management involves a continuous cycle of improvement and implementation (see Fig. 7.3).

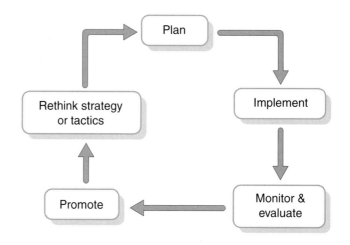

Figure 7.3 *Cycle of improvement and implementation*

As managers rarely get the chance to set up new departments and services from scratch, it is more usual to be in the midst of a continuous improvement cycle (described below).

Planning and implementation

When planning services for the future or improving current services offered, information managers need to be aware of customers' needs (explicit or implicit), resources available, environmental factors (e.g. what is permissible legally, new customer groups within the NHS, organizational demands) and value to the business or organization. Using this information, managers can start to formulate an information strategy.

Balancing all these factors, the manager and the team can start to define what services are worth implementing, define the workflow and processes and consider the team structure to fit the purpose (i.e. the tactics). Ideally this should be a cooperative process, with input and feedback from key customer groups and other stakeholders.

Having decided upon the strategy and tactics, implementation is the next stage, sometimes preceded by running a pilot scheme to test suitability for purpose. Successful implementation will depend upon good planning and organization, team involvement and leadership styles.

Service monitoring and evaluation

It is essential that any information service is monitored and evaluated. The information manager is held accountable for the services and their quality. Managers need to know that customers are satisfied, service quality is consistent and standards are met. Also, individual and team performance is enhanced when appropriately monitored and specific feedback given. Lastly, it is important to know the service dimensions in order to plan or justify resources and help promote the service.

Managers need to consider which services will be monitored and what the evaluation process will entail. An information department may offer a wide range of services, yet it may not be possible, expedient or necessary to monitor every service to the same degree. For example, enquiry handling within medical information departments is an important service and tends to be evaluated more closely than current awareness services.

There may already be evaluation methods available. AIOPI publishes *Guidelines on Standards in Medical Information* to cover some of the key services provided to external customers (Association of Information Officers in the Pharmaceutical Industry 1999). The

UK Drug Information Pharmacists Group (DIPG) has highly developed audit programmes to measure and monitor standards (Judd 1997).

Managers need to assess what they aim to achieve and thus which programme they need to implement. Many managers collect statistics on a monthly basis to monitor and report performance but may only run a customer satisfaction survey on an annual or infrequent basis. Inputs are very easy to measure (e.g. number of enquiries, information searches requested, articles ordered, journals checked in, promotional materials approved etc.). However it is outputs, costs, turnaround times and outcomes that are more useful management measures. Together, inputs and outputs can start to give some overall picture of quality.

Once the performance measures have been decided, the manager and team need to implement a programme. Methods can include:

- customer questionnaires
- telephone checks with customers
- ad hoc discussions with customers
- user group contacts
- focus groups
- peer review.

All these methods have their particular place, with advantages and disadvantages. Sarah Cook (1997) discusses customer surveys and their validity in some detail in her excellent book on customer care. As discussed above, both AIOPI and DIPG have designed audit programmes to use by medical or drug information departments. Research information departments are also keen to benchmark their services (see Chapter 10).

Feedback from customer surveys and other outcome measurements will therefore help the information manager to rethink tactics and possibly strategy too, further tailoring the service to customers' needs.

Service promotion

Information services have been shown to provide value to the organization. Unless customers are aware of these services and can make best use of them, their value to the organization may not be fully recognized.

Therefore it is important that any department promote the range and dimensions of the service. There are three methods that can be used: public relations (PR), marketing and advertising. In all three methods, the aim is to provide the right message to the right people at the right time in the right format. It is important to bear in mind that promotion is to individuals, not groups. One format will not fit all customers.

PR involves the use of third party endorsement to promote the service. The aim is to create favourable attitudes amongst the target audience using case studies, quotes or case histories. An example could be use of quotes from a few key customers within a product newsletter to motivate other customers. This will give the readers some more ideas of how to use the service to their advantage. Other third parties could be internal managers (e.g. product managers, research heads, hospital consultants), internal peers and external professionals. PR needs to be used in combination with advertising (e.g. a stand at the sales conference, business cards with freephone numbers, pens etc).

The next stage is to identify internal and external customers' needs, actual or potential. For a pharmaceutical industry medical information department, customers outside the company may include doctors, pharmacists, nurses, advisors, formulary committees, government bodies, associations, patient groups, etc. Internal customers include sales, marketing and medical departments. We can use various methods to tease out their expectations and needs, such as questionnaires and ad hoc discussions as outlined earlier.

When we know whom we want to target and what we want to say in order to promote our services, we need to choose an appropriate format. Examples may include bulletins, newsletters, media read by customers, face-to-face meetings, internet services and internal emails. The information we provide about our services needs to be tailored to customers' specific needs. For example, a bulletin written for a sales audience may be inappropriate to use for clinical research staff.

The results of promotional activities should be monitored to assess their effectiveness and to make improvements.

Further development areas for managers

Successful professionals take responsibility for their own learning. We choose to develop our skills and competencies to further our career goals, to improve our job performance, to acquire or develop specific skills or qualities and to achieve our own potential (self-actualization).

Whatever our job, it is important to consider the basic skills and qualities that are required and to identify personal development needs. Psychometric tests and self-assessment centres can help to give an independent view of our performance as managers and help us to identify development areas. Even simple tools such as a SWOT analysis can help to define our training needs. Use of the techniques described in Chapter 19 will provide a vehicle of development for most managers. The self-development book by Pedler et al (1994) makes a useful starting point and includes questionnaires to analyse further development areas and ways in which these needs can be addressed.

It has not been possible in this chapter to cover all of the areas that are relevant to the skills needed by information managers in the pharmaceutical industry or healthcare services. Some books for further reading are Buzan (1995), Fleming (1997), Richards (1998) and Russell-Jones (1995). I have found them useful, practical and readable, but they are just a small selection of the many available on these topics.

References

Adair J 1987 Effective teambuilding. Pan Books, London

Association of Information Officers in the Pharmaceutical Industry 1999 AIOPI guidelines on standards for medical information departments. http://www.aiopi.org.uk

Badenoch D, Reid C, Burton P, et al 1994 The value of information. In: Feeney M, Grieves M (eds) The value and impact of information. British Library Research Series, Bowker Sauer, London

Belbin R M 1996 Team roles at work. Butterworth Heinemann, Oxford

Blanchard K, Zigarmi P, Zigarmi D 1985 Leadership and the one minute manager. HarperCollins, London

Buzan T 1995 Use your head. BBC Books, London

Cook S 1997 Customer care. Kogan Page, London

Fleming I 1996 The teamworking pocketbook. Management Pocketbooks, Alresford

InPharm website address: www.inpharm.com. Accessed on 1st June 1999. Webmaster: Peter Llewellyn, InPharm.

Judd A (ed) 1997 UK drug information manual. UK Drug Information Pharmacists Group, Leeds

McBride J, Clark N 1996 20 steps to better management. BBC Books, London

Pease A 1997 Body language. How to read others' thoughts by their gestures. Sheldon Press, London

Pedler M, Burgoyne J, Boydell T 1994 A manager's guide to self development, 3rd edn. McGraw-Hill, London

Pharmiweb website address: www.pharmiweb.com. Accessed on 14th May 1999. Webmaster: Pharmiweb.

Russell-Jones N 1995 The managing change pocketbook. Management Pocketbooks, Alresford

Taylor R S 1986 Value-added processes in information systems. Ablex Publishing Corporation, New Jersey

Further Reading

Buzan T 1995 Use your head. BBC Books, London

Fleming I 1997 The time management pocketbook 4th edn. Management Pocketbooks, Alresford

Richards M 1998 The stress handbook. Management Pocketbooks, Alresford

Russell-Jones N 1995 The managing change pocketbook. Management Pocketbooks, Alresford

Chapter 8

Medicines information in the UK National Health Service

Alan Judd

Introduction

A review of UK drug information (DI) published in early 1999 (Hands et al 1999) described it as 'a hospital pharmacy specialist service whose emergence in 1969 coincided with an explosion in both the development of new drugs and literature related to them'. Before that time much pharmacy expertise was centred on the traditional skills of compounding, manufacturing and dispensing, with information on medicines coming from pharmacopoeias, formularies and the pharmaceutical industry. Pharmacists did provide pharmaceutical and clinical information on medicines but this was not identified as a key clinical role until the 1970s.

The establishment of DI services initially in London and Leeds in 1969 and then throughout the country over the next several years, plus the emergence of ward pharmacy, propelled hospital pharmacy into the clinical arena. These developments were stimulated by the Noel Hall Report in 1970 and by 1980 had been recognized and welcomed in the medical and pharmaceutical press (Anon 1978, Leach 1978) and by government (Jenkins 1979, Royal Commission 1979, Vaughan 1980).

New and potent drugs brought with them many patient benefits but also new problems of iatrogenic disease. The investigation of drugs' effectiveness and associated risks stimulated vast increases in published research, reviews and comments, all of which needed finding, collating and analysing before the information could be related to patient care. The traditional information resources mentioned previously were not up to this task and inherent problems with the potential for commercial bias in information from the pharmaceutical industry highlighted the need for clinically orientated non-biased information. DI services started to fulfil this role.

Structure

In the UK, the structure of DI services has mirrored the structure of the National Health Service (NHS). From the outset a tiered network was developed with larger regional centres working together to provide national coordination as well as supporting smaller local centres in their region. These local centres provide a service for the Trusts in which they are located and support primary care services in their vicinity. By 1992 there were 20 regional centres and over 200 local centres throughout the UK. NHS reorganizations have since decreased the number of regional centres but the number of local centres has continued to grow.

The reason for this structure is to provide, via a national network, a comprehensive countrywide service which is responsive to local needs but at the same time benefits from consistent and coordinated national standards, procedures and initiatives.

This whole network is coordinated by the UK Medicines Information Pharmacists Group (MIPG) which consists of the lead pharmacist from each regional centre but benefits increasingly from input by experienced drug information pharmacists from throughout the UK.

Aims and priorities

The aim of the UK DI service is to facilitate high quality patient care by the provision of accurate, timely, appropriate and unbiased information and advice on all aspects relating to the use of medicines.

This statement reflects goals and priorities which all DI services should bear in mind. It is not enough to make sure that information or advice is not wrong, it also has to be tailored to the particular situation (or patient); it must be there when needed and, as far as possible, it should be full, non-selective and non-biased. Bias can be a difficult element to eliminate and where that is not possible its presence needs always to be acknowledged.

In any new and developing role, achievement of a high quality service must be a priority but once systems are in place to facilitate this, other priorities begin to emerge. In the UK this meant that in the early days training, standards, procedures and audit were high priorities at a national level which led to the publication of a *UK Drug Information Manual* (Judd 1997). This continues to the present day and has been joined in recent years by high priority being given to work on evaluating and disseminating information on new drugs, the use of advances in information technology and the refocusing of NHS DI services to incorporate both primary and secondary care sectors. Important developments which provide new areas for DI services are NHS Direct and the emergence of Primary Care Groups/Trusts.

NHS Direct is a government-funded telephone-based service offering direct, free public access to specially trained nurses who can provide health information and advice at all times (Mason 1999). DI pharmacists are involved in training and supporting NHS Direct in both the development and continued functioning of the service.

Primary Care Groups /Trusts are NHS groups of doctors, nurses and other healthcare professionals who supply the primary care needs for a specific geographical area from a number of separate centres. Typically each group serves 50 000–100 000 patients and arranges for the provision of secondary healthcare for these patients. Pharmacists are involved as prescribing advisers and as such either provide a drug information service to their group or call upon DI centres to do so.

Role of drug information

A DI pharmacist in the NHS has three main roles. The first is that of a literature specialist with skills in expediting access to drug-related literature. The second is that of a specialist adviser with the principal function of enhancing the quality of patient care by providing information and advice based on carefully evaluated data. The third role is one of a trainer to help in providing pharmacists, clinicians and nurses with the appropriate skills in choosing and using medicines.

The spread of activities currently undertaken by UK DI illustrates these roles (Table 8.1). Enquiry answering forms a large part of the work of any DI service. It incorporates accessing the literature, collating, interpreting and evaluating the data and finally communicating these findings in a useful format. This process is helped by application of IT skills, access to appropriate resources and the development of specialists who can advise their colleagues in areas such as drug use in pregnancy, alternative medicine, liver and renal disease, paediatrics and mental health. An increasing amount of information is supplied proactively in the

Table 8.1 *Services provided by UK drug information centres*

Service	Description
Answering enquiries	Enquiries received from doctors, nurses, pharmacists, other healthcare professionals, patients and the public
Specialist information and advice	Drug use in: pregnancy, breastfeeding, dentistry, renal and hepatic disease, HIV/AIDS, poisoning, alternative medicines, travel, paediatrics, mental health, ophthalmology
Publications	Current awareness, prescribing advice, therapy reviews
Information on new drugs	From horizon scanning for drugs in development to reviews on newly marketed products
Support for drug and therapeutics committees	Information and advice in both primary and secondary care
Adverse drug reaction reporting	Coordination and collation
Data input to major databases	e.g. Pharmline, Micromedex
Education and training	For pharmacists, doctors, nurses and other healthcare professionals
Ward based clinical pharmacy	Carried out by the majority of DI pharmacists
Clinical trials/Ethics committees	Coordination of pharmacy involvement and membership of local research ethics committees

Adapted with permission from *UK DI Manual* 4th edn. (Judd 1997)

form of new drug evaluations, horizon scanning (the process of gathering and assessing information on potential medicinal drugs which are in their development stages prior to licensing and marketing), guidelines and other prescribing advice. The skills required for these roles are little different from those needed in enquiry answering, except perhaps with a greater emphasis on written rather than oral communication expertise.

Pharmacists working very closely with clinical teams need many of the skills once largely associated with DI; finding, evaluating and presenting information and advice is part of their daily work. Therefore, in many hospitals the DI pharmacist is now as much a trainer as a provider of information.

Resources (see also Chapter 2)

Resource considerations for DI cover the whole spectrum from buildings to paper clips and, most importantly, include the people who will deliver the service.

The exact nature of the resources used depends on the type of service being provided, but there are a number of factors common to all health service DI provision.

Environment

Good access is vital for any information service which answers enquiries. If contact with enquirers is to be face to face, then physical aspects such as convenient location, good signposting and consultation areas need to be given priority. If, however contact is mostly electronic, then the telephone system, facsimile and email assume greater importance.

Table 8.4
Recommended reference sources: drug interactions/adverse effects

Title	Authors/Editors	Publisher
Drug Interactions	Stockley	Pharmaceutical Press
Drug Interactions Analysis & Management	Hansten & Horn	Lea & Febiger
Meylers Side Effects of Drugs	Dukes, ed.	Excerpta Medica

Adapted with permission from *UK DI Manual*, 4th edn. (Judd 1997)

Table 8.5
Recommended reference sources: medicine and pharmacology

Title	Authors/Editors	Publisher
Applied Therapeutics: The Clinical Use of Drugs	Katcher et al	Applied Therapeutics
Clinical Pharmacology (or equivalent)	Laurence	Churchill Livingstone
Drug Prescribing in Renal Failure: Dosing Guidelines for Adults	Bennett et al	Am J Coll Phys (via BMJ Publications)
Drugs in Pregnancy and Lactation	Briggs et al	Williams & Wilkins
Herbal Medicine	Carol et al	Pharmaceutical Press
Interpretation of Diagnostic Tests	Wallach	Little, Brown
Merck Manual of Diagnosis and Treatment	Berkow, ed	Merck
Oxford Textbook of Medicine	Weatherall et al, eds	Oxford University Press
Goodman & Gilman's The Pharmacological Basis of Therapeutics (9th edn 1996)	Hardman et al, eds	McGraw-Hill
Special Tests: The Procedure and Meaning of Commoner Tests in Hospital	Evans	Mosby
Therapeutic Drugs	Dollery et al, eds	Churchill Livingstone
Wound Management and Dressings	Thomas	Pharmaceutical Press
The Renal Drug Handbook	Burn & Ashley, eds	Radcliffe Medical Press
Palliative Care Formulary	Twycross et al	Radcliffe Medical Press

Adapted with permission from *UK DI Manual*, 4th edn. (Judd 1997)

The sources listed in these tables are not the only ones which are found useful and larger DI centres or those with specialist services have access to many others. Commonly these include texts reflecting all the medical specialties as well as travel medicine, pharmacokinetics, medical statistics and clinical trials.

In spite of the advances in electronic data manipulation all UK DI services still maintain paper-based filing systems which contain manufacturers' literature, copies of journal articles, bulletins, drug reviews etc. A variety of methods are used to index such files but many are alphabetical and based on thesaurus terms from Pharmline (see Further Information).

Table 8.6
Recommended reference sources: journals

Title	Publisher
American Journal of Health-System Pharmacy	American Society of Hospital Pharmacy
Annals of Pharmacotherapy	DICP
British Medical Journal	British Medical Association
Drug and Therapeutics Bulletin	Consumers Association
Lancet	Elsevier
Medicine	Medical Education
Monthly Index of Medical Specialities (MIMS)	Haymarket Publishing
Pharmaceutical Journal	Pharmaceutical Press
Prescriber	A & M Publishing
Prescribers' Journal	The Stationery Office
Drugs	Adis International
Journal of the American Medical Association	American Medical Association
New England Journal of Medicine	The Massachusetts Medical Society
Annals of Internal Medicine	American College of Physicians and American Society of Internal Medicine

Adapted with permission from *UK DI Manual*, 4th edn. (Judd 1997)

Table 8.7
Recommended reference sources: databases

Title	Publishers
Pharmline	UK DIPG
Medline	National Library of Medicine
Drugdex	Micromedex
Cochrane Library	Update Software
Tictac	The Stationery Office
Iowa Drug Information System (IDIS)	University of Iowa, College of Pharmacy

The recent rapid advances in computer technology, especially networking (local area networks, the worldwide web), have revolutionized DI and it is now essential that such facilities are available in all centres. The rapid dissemination of information and communications between centres means that professional networking has been greatly enhanced. Reduction in work duplication can now more easily be achieved and sharing of expertise and knowledge is very much simpler.

Staff

All the 260 or so UK DI centres have a named pharmacist responsible for the service. The larger centres have a number of additional pharmacists. Staff levels depend on available financial resources, the enquiry workload and the extent to which the service has managed to develop in respect of, for example, proactive information provision, support for primary care, support for regional or national initiatives, formulary work and clinical trials. Nearly all DI pharmacists working in local centres will have some ward-based clinical commitment and some may only have 50% or less of their time to spend on drug information work. At regional level the situation is more varied and it is relatively common for senior personnel not to have a ward-based clinical commitment although the junior staff may. Shared posts with primary care responsibilities are also becoming much more common and recently similar arrangements with NHS Direct have started to emerge.

Staff who are not pharmacists are rare in drug information but they do exist. A handful of science graduates, senior technicians and a librarian or two work very successfully at various locations and potentially have much to contribute to future DI services.

Secretarial/clerical support is vital but very difficult to secure in many centres. The result is that pharmacists may spend their time doing work which is hard to justify on either a professional or financial basis.

Training

Undergraduate/postgraduate/pre-registration

The teaching of skills relevant to DI is not widespread at the undergraduate level, although some pharmacy degree courses do include communication skills and the use of various information sources.

It is usually in the context of pre-registration training that DI is first taught. The Royal Pharmaceutical Society of Great Britain pre-registration Competence-based Training Programme contains practical criteria relating to communication, provision of advice and guidance and use of information sources, all of which have obvious relevance to DI. Additional to these mandatory topics, most hospital-based pre-registration pharmacists receive practical training and some limited experience in the provision of drug information. The skills discussed in this chapter under the heading of in-service training are also often taught at a rudimentary level during the pre-registration year.

Postgraduate courses in clinical pharmacy usually contain some tuition on the use and evaluation of information sources, including clinical trial results, in relation to choosing and using appropriate medicines but systematic training often does not take place unless a DI module is one of the options.

Accredited postgraduate courses in purely health service DI do not exist but a distance learning course is being developed. The City University, London, runs a master's degree and diploma course in Pharmaceutical Information Management which deals with the subject from both a pharmaceutical industry and NHS perspective. This course has proved to be a useful adjunct to the continuing education of the NHS DI pharmacists who have taken it so far.

In-service

Since the beginning of nationally coordinated DI services in the UK training has been a priority. One of the first national initiatives was to organize training for staff at regional centres and then an annual residential training course for new DI pharmacists. This residential course, which has been running since the late 1970s, takes place two or three times each year and provides training in drug information skills for 50–80 pharmacists annually. The increasing recognition that skills such as enquiry answering, evaluating of clinical information, data manipulation and efficient use of information sources are important per se has meant that pharmacists with responsibilities outside DI have been attending the training courses in growing numbers. Table 8.8 shows a typical course programme.

Table 8.8 *Programme for national drug information training course*

Topic	Time	Comments
Enquiry answering and oral	2–3 h	Group-work and video communications
Databases	3–4 h	Group, plenary and practical experience
Medical statistics	1 h	Plenary lecture
Clinical trial design and evaluation	4 h	Group-work and discussion
Writing skills	2–3 h	Plenary lecture and training exercises
Drug advertising	1 h	Plenary lecture
Service provision topics	2 h	Group work and discussion

Although up to 80 pharmacists per year may receive training on the residential course many more need workplace training prior to their working in a DI centre. This is facilitated by the training programme specifically written for the purpose and made available in the *UK Drug Information Manual* (Judd 1997). It provides for the training of pre-registration pharmacists and pharmacists new to DI and aims to develop knowledge and practical competence in:

■ enquiry answering, including effective written and oral communication
■ local procedures
■ active information provision
■ specialist DI skills.

These aims are further detailed in associated objectives, broken down into discrete topics.

The training methods employed include test exercises, examples with discussion, background reading, audio-visual material, supervised activities and monitoring performance by means of self-assessment and trainer assessment. Where questions are set for the trainee to answer, a tutor's sheet is also provided to guide tutors in their assessments.

The training programme also draws upon the other sections of the *UK Drug Information Manual* to provide a basic awareness and initial training in:

■ management and resources
■ legal and ethical aspects of drug information
■ a review of information sources and use of databases
■ enquiry answering
■ evaluation of clinical trials
■ advertising and promotion of medicines
■ communications, oral and written
■ information on new drugs
■ the pharmaceutical industry
■ quality assurance programmes
■ risk management
■ information technology.

All of the topics in the training programme and those listed above are also classified as being suitable or not for higher level training of experienced pharmacists whose needs in this respect are equally as important as those of a new pharmacist.

Training for experienced pharmacists has centred around writing skills, use of technology, specialized areas of practice and general service issues such as ethics, standards and managing changes brought about by NHS reorganizations. Considerable expertise is needed to teach these subjects and finding suitably qualified people to do this can be quite a challenge. Many of these topics benefit from small group workshop-type tuition and this, plus the need to train 50–100 people has led us to provide sessions at the annual UK DI conference or repeated sessions at various locations around the country. Courses dealing with more strategic and management orientated issues are regularly organized for the most senior DI pharmacists who run large, often regional, services. These people need to be able to develop strategies to deal with change, review and develop standards and hone the skills necessary to move the national DI service forward.

Standards and quality assurance

Enquiry answering

The first standards to be developed were those relating to the resources (previously described in this chapter) and procedures which enable an enquiry answering service to operate at a professionally acceptable level. The standards cover access to the service, time taken to answer, the availability of suitably qualified staff, quality of the answer and meeting the needs of the enquirer. These can all be audited using the first UK DI audit programme which was introduced in 1990. This includes check lists and agreed criteria supplied to each DI centre. Examples of customer questionnaires and accompanying letters are also supplied to assist in the process.

To help in matching staff members to workload a time/activity matrix has been designed on which most DI tasks are listed together with their associated time requirements. For example a hospital-based DI service answering 1000 enquiries per year would need a minimum of a half a full-time pharmacist doing nothing other than answering enquiries. If other activities were undertaken, four hours would be needed for each copy of a newsletter, six hours would be needed for each drug and therapeutics new drug review and a minimum of 15 hours contact time for training each pre-registration student.

Continuing education

The second set of standards deals with continuing education and training. They are divided into three sections to accommodate pharmacists with varying levels of experience. Four separate standards covering the content of training programmes, who does the training, how much training is needed and when it is needed have been developed.

Publications

Drug information publications are the subject of the third set of standards. In a similar way to the other standards, aims are set out and then detailed procedures are given plus check lists of criteria so that quality assurance measures can be carried out in a uniform manner. The relevant elements under this heading are considered to be preparation of text, proofreading and checking procedures, legal considerations and copyright.

All three sets of standards are designed to ensure a uniformly high quality of service provided across the UK by suitably trained and knowledgeable staff. If service quality is found not to be acceptable at a particular time or in a particular place these standards also assist in identifying the reason for this and remedying the situation.

Standards are constantly being reviewed and revised in light of NHS developments and changing needs. Current areas for revision include non-pharmacists working in DI services, clinical governance and process quality in addition to output.

Risk management

Over the past few years risk management has been identified as important in many areas of pharmacy activity and drug information is no exception. The aim of risk management is the elimination of avoidable risk, the management of adverse incidents, reduction or elimination of harm to patients and the safeguarding of assets of all kinds. In the drug information setting a number of items (see Table 8.9) potentially contribute to this process in the UK and these have been set out in the DI manual so that all DI centres may use the central guidance to develop local risk management programmes.

Legal and ethical aspects of drug information (see also Chapter 17)

All pharmacists should be aware of the legal and ethical principles which govern the practice of their profession. Drug information, as a relatively new specialized function, has no UK case law. However, in recent years a code of practice and associated guidelines have been developed. These incorporate relevant sections from *Medicines, Ethics and Practice. A guide for pharmacists* (2000), published by the Royal Pharmaceutical Society, plus sections dealing with the items listed in Table 8.10.

The intention of these guidelines is to draw attention to those laws and regulations which govern our practice so that the legal pitfalls may be avoided. They are thus an integral part of risk management. For example it is very easy to fall foul of the copyright laws when the photocopier is so convenient and easy to use. If a service receives enquiries from patients or the public, where does the UK Data Protection Act affect us when these enquiries are documented and for how long do such documents need to be kept? Issues such as these can be difficult for any one service or individual but we hope the national guidelines produced by the Drug Information Pharmacists Group (Judd 1997) go some way to address these problems.

	Service element	Examples
Table 8.9 *Risk management factors*	Communications	Misunderstandings, confidentiality
	Staff	Poor selection, training, supervision
	Procedures	Failure to follow, none defined, poor documentation
	Environment	Lack of space, interruptions, noise
	Planning	Lack of, or poor quality
	Resources	Poor quality, not meeting standards
	Technical/professional expertise	Inadequate training, qualifications
	Organizational	Stress, conflict, poor recognition of risks
	Legal and ethical	Unlicensed drug use, copyright, conflict of interest

Adapted with permission from *UK DI Manual*, 4th edn, Update 1. (Judd 1997)

Sales representatives are among the most frequent users of medical information services. Medical information personnel should develop good teamwork with the sales representatives, providing them with the information, evidence and knowledge that they require to support their discussions with their customers. At the same time, the sales representatives need to understand the medical information department's role in giving a balanced view of the evidence on a subject. The medical information department is not there to 'sell' products but it does back up the representative by supplying the evidence in support of claims about efficacy and so on and by answering questions that doctors raise. As more emphasis is placed on evidence-based medicine (Sackett et al 1996), the value of effective information services supporting the sales effort will continue to grow.

Reviewing promotional materials

Materials such as advertisements, brochures, slide packs etc. that are used to promote the use of a company's products must comply with legal regulations and codes of practice (see Chapter 16). The medical information department in many companies (notably in the UK, though this is not always the case in other countries) has an important role in checking such materials before they are approved for use.

A proactive approach to reviewing promotional materials is helpful. The medical information and medical departments must check promotional materials to ensure that claims are accurate, valid, up to date and that they do not mislead. In doing this job there is always a risk of alienating the marketing or sales person who produced the item. He or she no doubt invested considerable time, effort and enthusiasm in the piece and may feel discouraged if inaccuracies or potential breaches of the relevant code of practice are pointed out. Imagine how a product manager would feel if the medical information department's comments about an item were: 'You cannot make that statement because it breaches clause X of the code of practice. The data shown in this graph are inaccurate and will have to be redrawn'.

If you are involved in checking promotional material you can contribute most by seeking a partnership approach. Instead of simply pointing out what is inaccurate or unacceptable, try to offer alternatives. Pharmaceutical promotion is most helpful when the claims that are made are well-substantiated and the product in question meets the prescriber's needs. By seeking to understand the promotional strategy and by proactively providing high quality information and advice to support it, you will be seen as part of the team that develops effective promotion. The marketing department for its part should actively encourage participation by the medical information department in developing promotional materials.

Competitor analysis

A pharmaceutical company should have up-to-date information on the medicines that are marketed or that are being developed by other companies. Therefore, the medical information department in a company will often provide analyses of products that compete with the company's own medicines. Good medical information skills in searching the literature, analysing data from clinical trials and synthesizing this information into a well-structured report or briefing provide an invaluable service to a company. It is also important to keep track of what is said about the company's medicines and competitors' products at congresses, in news reports, in market analysts' reports and through market research activities. The medical information function can play a role here by attending key congresses, monitoring newswires and other specialized sources (Mullen et al 1997) and through its links with the sales force.

More detailed analysis of competitor companies and their products may well be the role of a competitor analysis function or business information department.

Patient information

Patients are becoming increasingly knowledgeable about their conditions and their treatments. They also want and expect to receive more information about the medicines that they are taking. This can put the medical information department in a difficult position as it is often the main group within the company that deals with patients' enquiries and yet it may be restricted in the information that it can provide.

Article 3 of European directive 92/28/EEC on the advertising of medicinal products for human use states: 'Member States shall prohibit the advertising to the general public of medicinal products which are available on prescription only . . .'. This does not mean that medical information departments may not provide information about medicines to patients or other members of the public if they request it. It is certainly permissible to provide factual information about a medicine. However, unless the medical information professional understands the patient's level of knowledge there is a risk of being too simplistic and appearing to patronize or, conversely, of blinding the patient with science. Usually in a telephone conversation it is possible to gain a reasonable idea of what the patient knows already and what information will be most helpful. However, a patient may also be so knowledgeable that the person dealing with the enquiry assumes that he or she is a health professional! Thus, always ask, discreetly, who the enquirer is and the reason for the enquiry.

Medical information staff may believe that their company's policy or local regulations or codes of practice prevent them from providing anything but the most basic information to patients. This need not be the case and, if in doubt, it is worth discussing policy with company management and with the pharmaceutical industry's association (the ABPI in the UK). Colleagues in medical information departments in other companies may also be prepared to describe their approach. Much misinformation about medicines is now all too easily available to patients through the internet and other media and it is important that companies have the opportunity to provide factually accurate and helpful information.

Since 1995 EPARs (European Public Assessment Reports) have been issued for products that have received Marketing Authorisations through the European Agency for the Evaluation of Medicinal Products (EMEA). Copies are openly available on the internet at the EMEA website (http://www.emea.eu.int). In the USA, Summary Basis of Approval reports are available to patients. Both types of documents provide useful though rather technical information about new medicines.

Companies produce product information leaflets (PILs), which are written specifically for patients. They are intended to provide brief details about the medicine, its uses and its safety in an easy to read format. PILs are not, by their nature, very detailed and may be too superficial for knowledgeable patients.

In dealing with requests from patients, the doctor-patient relationship must always be borne in mind. Usually the patient should be recommended to speak to his or her doctor if advice is needed about a personal medical matter.

Pharmacovigilance

Some medical information departments have an active role in collecting and following up reports of adverse events associated with the company's products. Many companies have separate pharmacovigilance or safety departments, but the medical information department may still be the first point of contact for doctors, pharmacists or even patients when reporting adverse events. Medical information personnel must be aware of the legal requirements and relevant timelines about reporting such events to the appropriate authorities. Further information on this subject is provided in Chapter 12.

which are complex. Many go unanswered and yet 'most of the questions generated by doctors can be answered, usually from electronic sources, but it is time consuming and expensive to do so – *and demands information skills that many doctors do not have*' (our italics). Very importantly, doctors often want more than just information—they want support, guidance, judgement and feedback.

As identified in both of these studies, health professionals want easy access to information. More than that, they want access to knowledge, advice and guidance. Medical information departments can help meet these needs by ensuring that:

- health professionals know about the services that they provide and how to contact the department
- procedures are in place to deal with enquiries efficiently
- personnel are adequately trained and have detailed knowledge of the subjects with which they deal.

Despite Smith's comment that most questions can be answered from electronic sources, we are still a long way from advanced computer intelligence to rival the skills and knowledge of a human expert. Moreover, computerized information systems have contributed to information overload as well as providing ways to cope with it. For many health professionals the problem is not lack of information but a need to find the most relevant information quickly and easily and then to distil the key facts and evidence from it. It has been said (Jewell 1988) that if you were to read one medical article every day, by the end of one year there would be 55 centuries' worth of articles remaining to be read! This can be a major challenge and knowledge may not be kept up to date, as Wyatt has pointed out regarding the treatment of hypertension: 'the strongest predictor of the drugs they prescribed was the doctor's year of qualification' (Wyatt 1991).

The evidence-based medicine movement has made much progress in recent years in producing systematic reviews that summarize up-to-date evidence about healthcare interventions (Bero & Rennie 1995). No matter how comprehensive in coverage such systematic reviews of the published literature become, there will continue to be a need for easy access to other, sometimes unpublished, information and to knowledge and expertise.

Medical information departments can provide a crucial role in helping health professionals. They have access to the available information about particular medicines and related subject areas. They have the skills to find the specific information that their customers need. Most importantly, they usually have detailed knowledge about the medicines that they deal with and they have access, when needed, to the company's experts.

Medical information staff must also strive to meet the particular needs of their customers in their marketing and sales departments in the ways outlined earlier. To do their job well, medical information personnel must understand the company's marketing and sales strategies. Ideally, they should be providing information and knowledge to help develop those strategies. Instead of waiting to be asked for information, they should actively provide information to their marketing and sales colleagues. They can do this through, for example, news alerts and participation in planning and strategy meetings. In order to be accepted as team members with marketing and sales staff they must show that their contributions add value. In particular, they must advertise successes. Examples might include:

- the inclusion of a new medicine in a formulary as a result of information supplied by the medical information department
- information and ideas contributed to a marketing plan or promotional campaign for a product
- financial savings made by writing a product monograph or other material in-house rather than employing an external agency
- training sales representatives and other staff about a new product
- positive feedback from external customers about the value of information provided.

Medical information personnel must promote the value of their services. Nobody else will do this for them!

Adding value: information and knowledge management

The previous section emphasized the importance of medical information personnel understanding their customers' needs and proactively providing information when appropriate before it is requested.

The usefulness of an information service depends on the value of the information provided and on the impact that the information has, as well as on other factors such as speed. A number of authors have described the progression from data to information to knowledge and even to wisdom (Davenport & Prusak 1998, Slawson et al 1994, Taylor 1994). In this progression, data may be considered to be individual facts or numerical values, information is organized data, 'the meaning we assign to facts' (Slawson et al 1994), and knowledge is information that has been analysed and understood. Wisdom is the 'possession of experience and knowledge together with the power of applying them critically or practically' (Concise Oxford Dictionary). Value is added as data are converted to information and then to knowledge leading to action, decision-making or planning. An information service adds value by providing not simply data but structured information and, better still, evaluated information or knowledge.

There has been much discussion in recent years about knowledge management. See for example Davenport & Prusak (1998) and Stewart (1997). Through the activities of evaluating information, synthesizing information into summaries of what is known about a particular subject, and by sharing knowledge and expertise, the medical information function plays a very important role in knowledge management (Robson et al 1999). There is further discussion about knowledge management in Chapter 4.

Standards and performance measures in medical information

High standards are essential in a medical information service. Information provided to healthcare professionals about medicines and other treatments can have significant effects on patients' welfare and safety (Marshall 1994).

The Code of Practice for Drug Information Services in the UK National Health Service states that the aim of drug information services is 'to promote the safe, effective and economic use of medicinal products in patients by the active and passive provision of accurate drug information and advice' (Judd 1997). A key part of the role of a company's medical information department is to provide accurate and relevant information to healthcare professionals to aid them in the appropriate use of medicines.

As is the case for any other professional activity, quality assurance of medical information services is important to ensure that appropriate standards are set in line with customers' needs, and that performance is evaluated.

Standards

In the UK, AIOPI has established guidelines on standards for medical information departments (Association of Information Officers in the Pharmaceutical Industry 1999).

In brief, the guidelines cover the following:

- Access to the medical information service—Companies must have a dedicated resource (normally the medical information department) to deal with medical enquiries.

Quality

The quality of an information service may be assessed by audit. Ideally, auditing should be carried out by a third party from outside the department, such as a medical adviser or the medical director, but this may not be possible.

For a quality audit a sample of the department's outputs should be considered, including responses to enquiries, literature searches and current awareness bulletins. The auditor should assess a number of factors such as:

- how far did each response address the question that had been asked (or did it miss the point or include information that was not relevant)?
- what sources of information were used to answer the question and were any important sources missed?
- were records kept of literature searches that were carried out?
- was an appropriate search strategy used in each case?
- was the information provided accurate, up to date and a fair summary of the available evidence?
- is the information provided in current awareness bulletins up to date and is it presented in an effective way (is it easy to read, does it draw the reader to key issues, is there analysis of these issues etc.)?

There is no one 'right way' of performing an audit, but it is important that a meaningful assessment of the quality of a department's services is carried out periodically.

Customer satisfaction

A quality audit will provide information on the standards to which an information department operates but in itself it will reveal nothing about the degree to which the department's services meet customers' needs. Customer feedback is essential if the department is to demonstrate that it is providing worthwhile services and if the department is to develop those services appropriately. Feedback may be spontaneous, or it may be solicited informally during conversations with customers or formally through structured questionnaires and surveys. All feedback is valuable but structured feedback is especially useful as it can provide information on the needs of groups of customers and how well or otherwise the department's services meet those needs.

AIOPI has produced a simple questionnaire that may be modified or used as is to solicit feedback from customers of medical information departments. Customers should not be bombarded with frequent questionnaires and medical information departments need to remember that departments from other companies may be sending their own questionnaires to the same people. In the UK, AIOPI has been working with the UK Drug Information Pharmacists' Group to agree to ways of using questionnaires without overwhelming pharmacists and other healthcare professionals with frequent mailings. Further information and a copy of the AIOPI questionnaire may be obtained from the AIOPI website—http://www.aiopi.org.uk/standards.htm.

Impact

As essential as feedback on customer satisfaction is, it may not provide information about the effectiveness or impact of medical information services. Such information can be crucially important when justifying the continued existence or development of services. Appropriate customers need to be asked how the medical information department's services help them. Find out whether information provided has led to specific actions, decisions or plans and if so what the consequences were. Sales representatives may confirm that information supplied has led to the inclusion of a medicine in a formulary, thus directly contributing to sales; such evidence is very valuable when arguing for increased (or even continued) funding of medical information services.

Marshall (1994) described a particularly interesting study of the impact of information services. A survey among 208 hospital physicians in the New York area revealed that information provided by hospital libraries had led to changes in advice to patients, drug treatment and diagnosis, and it led to reductions in surgery and in the length of hospital stay. Most importantly of all, the physicians reported that the information they had received helped them to reduce patient mortality. It is reasonable to believe that the information provided by medical information departments can have a similar impact on patients' well-being, but departments will need to find the evidence.

Financial measures

Reference has already been made to the possible contribution of medical information services to sales of a company's products. It is also important to compare the costs of the department's services with those of alternatives and to consider ways in which the department can save money for the company.

For example, the department may save substantial amounts from the marketing department's expenditure by writing monographs, brochures, formulary packs and so on that would otherwise be outsourced to an agency. If the medical information department writes such materials it may be able to cross-charge marketing and other departments for the work. In this way the information department could become self-financing.

Efficient departments will constantly be looking for ways of improving their operations. Process improvements may lead to reduced costs.

The future

It has been suggested (many times over many years!) that the future is bleak for information professionals. When CD-ROM versions of databases such as Medline first appeared users claimed that they were so user-friendly that there would be no need for skilled intermediaries to perform literature searches—non-skilled searchers would apparently be able to search just as effectively. The personal computer was going to replace information professionals because users would be able to find all the information they needed at the touch of a few keys. Then, the internet would give everyone more or less instant access to all the information they could possibly want and, with the advent of push technology, they would receive up-to-the-minute news on the subjects of interest to them. More recently still, call centres and companies that provide answering services (Felton & Leeuw 1998) would reputedly be able to do everything that a medical information department does but presumably more efficiently.

As the concept of knowledge management has developed, it has at last been recognized that information technology by itself is just a tool. 'It is patently the case . . . that many businesses have computerised everything in sight but have not found commensurate improvements in their effectiveness' (Davies 1994).

An information-intensive industry such as the pharmaceutical industry will continue to need the skills of information professionals, but medical information staff must ensure that their companies understand their role, the skills they have and the value that they can provide. Medical information personnel must be recognized as professionals, and here it is pertinent to consider what we mean by a professional: 'The true professional commands a body of knowledge—a discipline that must be updated constantly' (Quinn et al 1996). From all that has been said earlier about the activities of medical information departments and their standards, it should be clear that the staff of those departments perform professional roles. Yet too often (or so it seems to these authors), the skills of those staff are not understood within their companies. One of us (AR) remembers some years ago a former medical director saying that he wanted to spend an hour or two learning how to search databases. As if 'an hour or two' would be enough to gain an adequate understanding of the structures of even a few key databases and the necessary skills to search them well.

Important though the traditional skills of searching for and finding information are, we believe that the value added by information professionals as knowledge workers is more important still. 'Unlike information intermediaries, whose main function is to search, knowledge workers use searching as a means to an end' (Feldman 2000). The real value is added by analysing and interpreting information, building and sharing knowledge to answer questions and to aid decision-making and planning.

Those of us involved in medical information must remember the importance of promoting ourselves as professionals who perform a key role. We must find effective ways of demonstrating the value that we add through the various responsibilities outlined in this chapter. For the right people the future is bright with opportunities:

> *... the success of a corporation lies more in its intellectual and systems capabilities than in its physical assets. The capacity to manage human intellect—and to convert it into useful products and services—is fast becoming the critical executive skill of the age.* (Quinn et al 1996)

Medical information skills are indeed critically important for a successful pharmaceutical company.

References

Abbott C 1994 Performance measurement in library and information services. Aslib, London

Association of Information Officers in the Pharmaceutical Industry 1999 AIOPI guidelines on standards for medical information departments. Association of the British Pharmaceutical Industry London http://www.aiopi.org.uk

Bero L, Rennie D 1995 The Cochrane Collaboration. Preparing, maintaining, and disseminating systematic reviews of the effects of health care. Journal of the American Medical Association 274: 1935–1938

Colvin C L 1990 Understanding the resources and organisation of an industry-based drug information service. American Journal of Hospital Pharmacy 47: 1989–1990

Core Research Ltd 1999 Core resources of healthcare information, 1st edn. Core Research Ltd, Alton, Hampshire, UK

Davenport T H 1994 Saving IT's soul: human-centered information management. Harvard Business Review 72(2): 119–131

Davenport T H, Prusak L 1998 Working knowledge. Harvard Business School Press, Boston

Davies H 1994 Information and industry. In: ? eds The value of information to the intelligent organisation. University of Hertfordshire Press, Hatfield, ch 1, pp 13–14

Dollery C (ed), 1999 Therapeutic drugs, 2nd edn. Churchill Livingstone, Edinburgh

Feldman S 2000 The answer machine. Searcher 8(1): 58–79

Felton A, Leeuw M 1998 The medical communications centre—make or buy? Pharmaceutical Times June: 30–32

Gretz M, Thomas M 1995 The in-house database—nicety or necessity? Drug Information Journal 29: 161–169

Hopkins F, Galligher C, Levine A 1999 Medical affairs and drug information practices within the pharmaceutical industry: results of a benchmarking survey. Drug Information Journal 33: 69–85

Hull P 1996 Pharmaceutical published literature databases: a survey. Medical Reference Services Quarterly 15: 77–88

Huntingford A L, O'Callaghan R, Taylor J, et al 1990 A survey of industry medical information departments' activities. Pharmaceutical Journal 245: 238–239

Jewell D 1988 Reading scientific articles, or how to cope with the overload. Practitioner 232: 720–725

Judd A (ed) 1997 UK drug information manual 4th edn. UK Drug Information Pharmacists Group (Available from: Drugs and Poisons Information Service, The General Infirmary, Great George Street, Leeds LS1 3EX, UK.)

Malone P M, Mosdell K W, Kier K L, et al 1996 Drug information: a guide for pharmacists. Appleton & Lange, Stamford, Connecticut

Manifold C, Erkkila D M, Johnson C, et al 1998 The development of performance standards for medical communications personnel. Drug Information Journal 32: 1093–1107

Marshall J 1994 The impact of information services on decision-making: some lessons from the financial and health care sectors. In: Feeney M, Grieves M (eds) The value and impact of information. Bowker Saur, London ch 5, pp 195–211

Morton L T, Godbolt S (eds) 1992 Information sources in the medical sciences. Bowker Saur, London

Mullen A, Blunck M, Kalbfleisch E, et al 1997 Assessment, from an industrial user perspective, of some major competitor information files on pharmaceutical development projects. Journal of Information Science 23: 9–23

Parfitt K (ed) 1999 Martindale, the complete drug reference, 32nd edn. The Pharmaceutical Press, London

Pickering W R (ed) 1989 Information sources in pharmaceuticals. Bowker Saur, London

Quinn J B, Anderson P, Finkelstein S 1996 Managing professional intellect: making the most of the best. Harvard Business Review 74(2): 71–80

Rawn P. Hoffman-La Roche Ltd 1999 Drug Information & Safety Department survey of customer needs and satisfaction. Drug Information Journal 33: 525–539

Riggins J L, Ferguson K J, Miller S I, et al 1999 Globalizing medical information services at Eli Lilly and Company. Drug Information Journal 33 515–524

Robson A S, Blake J, Chandler R, et al 1996 Medical information services in the pharmaceutical industry: a survey of pharmacists' views with recommendations. Pharmaceutical Journal 256: 864–866

Robson A, Bandle E, Ince J 1999 Medinfolink: a practical approach to knowledge management at SmithKline Beecham Pharmaceuticals. In: Online Information 99, Proceedings. Learned Information Europe, Oxford, pp 187–191

Sackett D L, Rosenberg W C, Muir Gray J A, et al 1996 Evidence based medicine: what it is and what it isn't. British Medical Journal 312: 71–72

Shaughnessy A F, Slawson D C 1996 Pharmaceutical representatives. British Medical Journal 312: 1494

Slawson D C, Shaughnessy A F, Bennett J H 1994 Becoming a medical information master: feeling good about *not* knowing everything. Journal of Family Practice 38: 505–513

Smith R 1996 What clinical information do doctors need? British Medical Journal 313: 1062–1068

Stewart T A 1997 Intellectual capital, the new wealth of organisations. Nicholas Brealey Publishing, London

Sylvan L, Palmer-Shelvin N 1995 Bristol-Myers Squibb drug information department services. Hospital Pharmacy 30(1): 38–9, 44

Taylor R 1994 Value-added processes in information systems. Ablex Corporation Norwood, New Jersey

Thomas M, Gretz M 1996 From serum cholesterol in elephants to morbidity in Nepal: an empirical analysis of 6,729 on-line searches at Boehringer Mannheim GmbH. Drug Information Journal 30: 217–236

Vercellesi L, Miranda G F, Beretta A 1996 Drug information professionals and medical writers: an Italian view. Drug Information Journal 30: 891–895

Wyatt J 1991 Use and sources of medical knowledge. Lancet 338: 1368–1373

Yamamoto M, Onaka Y, Hirai T, et al 1995 Drug information in the Japanese pharmaceutical industry: analysis of an eight-year investigation. Drug Information Journal 29: 1201–1209

Further Reading

Ascione F J, Manifold C C, Parenti M A 1994 Principles of drug information and scientific literature evaluation. Drug Intelligence Publications, Hamilton, Illinois

Spilker B 1994 Multinational pharmaceutical companies: principles and practices, 2nd edn. Raven Press, New York

Chapter 10

Research information in the pharmaceutical industry

Elisabeth Goodman, with contributions from Jane Whittall and Debbie Morrison

Introduction

The Research and Development (R&D) process for a new medicine consists of all the steps from discovery, through development, to the point where the product is ready to go to market.

The focus of this chapter is on the research information needed to support the process, and how we, as information professionals, can help to influence that process to minimize the cycle time, and optimize the chances of a new chemical entity making it all the way to market.

The place of information services in research and development in the pharmaceutical industry

The R&D process—time and cost (see Fig. 10.1)

The challenges which the R&D scientist faces are multiple.

How to increase the speed of the whole process so that the time left on patent is optimized

One week can make a difference of as much as $11m loss in revenue for a big selling drug (Anon 1996). With the increased competition from generic medicines, patent life expiry can mean a loss of at least 50% of sales in the first year off patent. Development time takes anywhere between 10 and 16 years. The Centre for Medicines Research quotes a mean figure of 10–12 years (Lumley 1995).

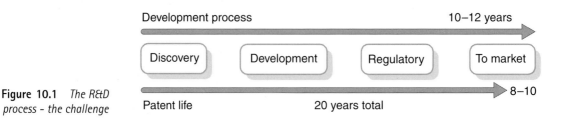

Figure 10.1 *The R&D process - the challenge*

How to increase the success rate, i.e. the proportion of compounds that achieve final new chemical entity (NCE) status

Typical figures quoted are only 1 in 10–20 000 compounds meeting that target, while the overall cost for getting one drug to market currently averages between $400 and $600 million.

How to increase the number and novelty of compounds made

With the continued trend in mergers and acquisitions in the pharmaceutical industry, companies in the top 10 would need to generate NCEs at the rate of two per year to ensure 5% growth over the next 10 years. However, the number of new molecular entities (NMEs) introduced on the world market decreased significantly over the past decade. A total of 176 company groups were responsible for marketing the 465 NMEs first launched between 1986 and 1995. Only six of these achieved the industry target of one or more per year, with the majority marketing only one NME over the 10 year period (Ashton 1996).

Components of the R&D process; maximizing the chances of success

The disciplines concerned

To put this chapter into context, we shall start with a simple overview of the component steps and disciplines in the R&D process (Fig. 10.2). This summary is derived (with amendments) from *A Textbook of Drug Design and Development* (Williams & Nadzan 1991), which also includes some useful examples. Although specific examples and applications of research information will not be highlighted until later in this chapter, you should, as you read this description of the R&D process, begin to recognize all the occasions when the work of an information professional might be of value.

For the last 100 years, the 'lock and key' hypothesis has acted as the main focus for compound design and drug targeting. The 'lock' may be a receptor for hormones, neurotransmitters or neuromodulators, the drug target then being an agonist that mimics the effects of these 'keys', or an antagonist that blocks their actions.

This simplistic view is being challenged by advances in our understanding of the mechanism of drug action. For instance, drugs may function as inhibitors of enzymes by acting as false substrates, or as cofactors which can modulate the catalytic process. Information from human genome sequencing has also had a major impact, affording numerous possibilities for potential drug targets and an increased understanding of the molecular basis of disease.

The medicinal chemist relies on receptor binding technology as a means of rapidly and cost-effectively deriving structure-activity relationships (SARs) for a series of related substructures or homologues at a given receptor or enzyme target. SARs thereby improve the ability to design compounds which better fit the target site.

As the efficacy of binding is not necessarily a true indication of desired activity, biochemists and pharmacologists supplement SARs with a range of functional assays. Biochemists may measure the change induced in a receptor-linked second messenger system, or the enzyme-related appearance or disappearance of products and substrates. Tissue assays may be used to monitor physiological effects such as muscle contraction or effects of blood sugar levels.

Pharmacologists undertake animal studies for the function of the desired drug target, and investigate effects on animal models of the disease.

In assessing the in vivo activities of these potential new chemical entities, it is important to demonstrate a correlation between drug efficacy and the actual absorption, presence or availability of the parent compound or its metabolites in plasma. The ultimate elimination

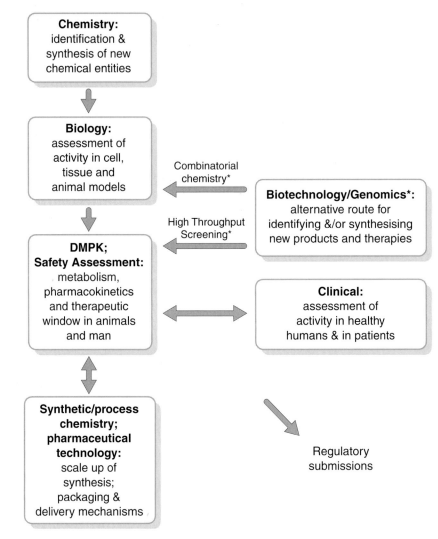

Figure 10.2 *Steps in the R&D process*

of the compound and metabolites also needs investigation. This absorption, distribution, metabolism, excretion (ADME) information will help to establish the ultimate drug vehicles, routes of administration and dose regimens to be used.

Safety assessment studies, both in vitro and in animal models, are used to assess the effects of the compound on bacterial and mammalian cell replication, on reproduction, immune systems and behaviour. Through these studies a therapeutic window can be established, i.e. the optimum effective dose with the minimal toxicological risk.

Clinical development consists of four phases, used to test the effectiveness and safety of the compound in humans.

- Phase I consists of studies in healthy human volunteers, with rising doses via the chosen route of administration. Drug metabolism and bioavailability studies are carried out at this time, and side-effects monitored. Some patients may also be included in these trials.
- Phase II trials continue to evaluate the safety of the compound and begin to monitor its efficacy in the selected patient population. This phase is divided into two stages: IIa is a limited trial; IIb is more broad range. During both stages the investigators are usually seeking biochemical indicators of drug efficacy.

■ Phase III is a full-scale, multicentre evaluation of the treatment in a large patient population. The dosage used in this stage is critical as the data from these trials form the basis of regulatory authority decisions.

■ Phase IV trials are used to monitor additional uses for a new drug for any subsequent NDA (new drug application).

Throughout the later stage testing of the compound in drug metabolism and pharmacokinetics (DMPK), safety assessment and clinical studies, chemists will be examining alternative, faster, more cost-effective routes for synthesizing and purifying the active chemical components. Effective large-scale synthetic routes need to be identified, and stable formulations derived for the ultimate dosage schedule selected.

Maximizing the chances of success

As mentioned above, the challenge for R&D is three-fold: to reduce the overall cycle time, to optimize the chances of success, and to maximize the number and novelty of potential new chemical entities.

Three key activities in the discovery phase of research that are helping to meet this challenge are: biotechnology, bioinformatics and genomics; combinatorial chemistry; high-throughput and 'smart' screening.

■ Biotechnology has traditionally been used in the pharmaceutical industry as an alternative method of synthesizing new drugs by using recombinant DNA technology to make biological end-products. However, the amount of information being generated from the human genome sequencing project has led to the emergence of bioinformatics as a new discipline at the interface of biology and computing. Bioinformatics provides the organizational and analytical computing tools required to extract the maximum value from biological sequence information. The huge effort in the genomics area has led to the identification of many new potential drug targets. Further down the discovery pipeline, genomic information can be used to identify individuals for whom a drug might not be suitable, thus reducing failure in clinical trials. (See also Cole & Bawden 1996.)

■ Medicinal chemists traditionally go about the process of identifying potential new chemical leads through structure-activity relationships. They gain as much mechanistic understanding as they can of the target receptor or enzyme site, identify a pharmacophore (a core structure which is shown to bind to and/or have activity at the site). They then synthesize variations of this pharmacophore until a compound with optimum activity is found. This process is slow and open to risk from competitors who may either reach the solution first, or who may have overlapping patent coverage.

Many companies complement such structured synthetic efforts by serendipitous screening of accumulated stocks of compounds over a range of assays. Another approach is to collect potential compounds from various natural product sources such as fermentation or microbes, plants and marine life (Williams & Nadzan 1991). Combinatorial chemistry combines the serendipity of these approaches with that of SAR. Through solid-phase chemistry, and the use of computers and robotics, whole libraries of related compounds are made at one time. These are, in turn, put through high-throughput screens for the rapid identification of potential leads. The medicinal chemist then isolates any particularly interesting compounds for further synthetic efforts or direct submission for more detailed screening.

■ As already alluded to, the concept of high-throughput screening is that of putting a large number of compounds through an array of computer operated screens. The aim is, through serendipity, to pick up potential leads which might either have been missed through more systematic approaches or arrived at more slowly. 'Smart' screening implies a more focused, but still large-scale variation of this approach.

The focus of the development phases of R&D has generally been to screen potential lead compounds and eliminate those which by reason of effectiveness, bioavailability or safety are not viable. Structure-activity models are not as easy to derive in these disciplines as in those for discovery. The main challenge has been to make the development processes as fast as possible. Pharmaceutical companies have for instance tried different models for R&D such that studies run in parallel rather than sequentially. Or they have sought ways of increasing the sophistication of the development studies so that non-viable compounds are rejected as soon as possible, thereby not wasting valuable R&D resources. The Centre for Medicines Research has reported on the expenditure by 44 leading companies on different phases of R&D in 1993 (Anon 1995). Discovery, including absorption, distribution, metabolism and excretion (ADME), accounted for 28% of expenditure. Toxicology and other kinetic tests in animals accounted for 10%, premarketing clinical evaluation 28.5%, postmarketing studies 10.5% and all other R&D activities other than discovery 23%.

However, Smith et al 1996 argue that considerable advances have been made in recent years such that basic rules can now be applied, particularly in the areas of absorption, distribution and elimination, to predict the behaviour of a drug based on its physicochemistry and structure. They argue that the combination of pharmacokinetics and pharmacodynamics at the discovery stage can lead to drugs with optimum performance characteristics.

The value/impact of research information

The most striking demonstration of the value/impact of research information in an R&D environment was reported by Koenig in 1990. The library and information environment of the four most highly productive US-based pharmaceutical companies was compared with that of the four least productive companies of comparable size (in terms of R&D budget). The output measure for productivity was the number of good new drugs developed. The more productive group of companies was on average three and a half times more productive than the less productive group.

The more productive companies were characterized by:

- greater openness to outside information
- rather less concern with protecting proprietary information
- greater information systems development effort
- greater end-user use of information systems and more encouragement of browsing and serendipity
- greater technical and subject sophistication of the information services staff
- relative unobtrusiveness of managerial structure and status indicators in the R&D environment.

An econometric indication of value was demonstrated by Moony & Oppenheim (1994). British industry spent £1080m +/- £474m in 1992 on patents and patent information. These figures include expenditure on obtaining intellectual property rights, maintaining and using products and services to find patent information when needed, and ensuring that staff have the necessary education to participate in the intellectual property process.

The concept of data mining is an illustration of the perceived value of information to the pharmaceutical industry. Data mining is the process of discovering meaningful new correlations, patterns and trends by sifting through large amounts of data stored in repositories, using pattern recognition technologies and statistical and mathematical techniques. These relationships might not otherwise be obvious to the human analyst. The retail, financial and medical sectors have so far led the way in getting results from this technology. Other examples are more sparsely distributed in manufacturing, chemical, petroleum, insurance, security and environmental sectors (Block 1995). However:

new trends in drug discovery are demanding a new level of integration between information systems used in all phases of research. This integration includes the requirement for analytical tools at the desktop that can be used by a range of researchers. When combined with the power of today's modern chemical database systems, these analysis tools offer new applications possibilities by allowing chemists to uncover important information stored in their data sets. By using modern computing methods for parallel computing, client-server capabilities, and analysis on large volumes of data, the mining of information from databases has considerably broader applications in the drug discovery process. (Morrell 1996)

Role and activities of research information departments

Research information, and information professionals in particular, have a role throughout the R&D process in providing scientists with the tools and services to obtain and manage external and internal information, both for the more traditional approaches to the R&D process, and in the exploitation of new technologies for maximizing their chances of success. In the next section of this chapter I will attempt to document the information inputs and outputs in the R&D process. Before doing this, it is worth noting the following challenges in R&D which effective information management can help to address:

- generating new leads
- understanding disease mechanisms
- identifying targets for cure or prevention
- developing effective models of the diseases
- sophisticated screening techniques
- minimizing use of animals
- sophisticated analysis techniques
- efficient drug synthesis techniques
- attractive and effective formulation.

In today's environment, the role of research (and development) information is to provide:

- current awareness (proactive) literature and patent services
- retrospective (reactive) literature and patent search services
- competitive information throughout the drug discovery and development process
- integration of information support into R&D project teams
- provision of end-user training/support and end-user databases
- access to full-text information via electronic journals and document delivery
- management/integration of internal chemical and biological information

Information flow in the R&D process: inputs and outputs

The information generated and used in the course of the R&D process is summarized in Figure 10.3. For each of these types of information input and output, there are new trends emerging in information management.

- 'Discussions with colleagues' are at the forefront of the knowledge sharing promoted by knowledge management: involving reassertion of the role of information professionals as members of R&D project and other teams. As members of such teams, information professionals will be much more attuned to the information requirements of their customers, and so can provide a more focused and timely information service. Other forms of knowledge sharing involve the promotion of groupware and intranet discussion forums, and more effective management of conference attendance and use of associated information.

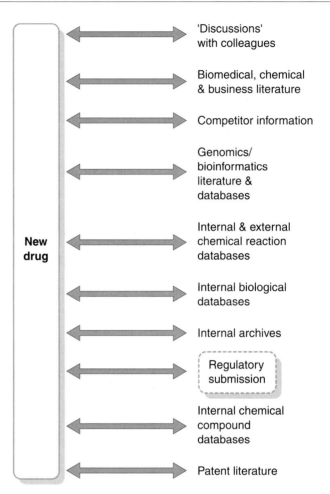

New drug

'Discussions' with colleagues

Biomedical, chemical & business literature

Competitor information

Genomics/ bioinformatics literature & databases

Internal & external chemical reaction databases

Internal biological databases

Internal archives

Regulatory submission

Internal chemical compound databases

Patent literature

Figure 10.3
Information inputs and outputs

- Patent, biomedical, chemical, business literature. The role of the information professional must be to influence the design of web-based and other sources for ever more friendly user front-ends, which require the minimum learning for effective use. At the same time, more sophisticated current awareness/alerting tools are also emerging such that users can again have the latest relevant information delivered to their desks or desktops. As described in Chapter 15, the result for information professionals is that we can now focus on providing real value-added responses to our customers' queries.

- Specialist skills are required to search chemical and genomic patent information sources effectively. The information professional has a crucial role to play in patent searching. Before any resources are expended in discovery, the field of investigation must be checked for competitor company or other patents. Existing patents covering the scope of the proposed area of investigation would seriously limit the scope for commercial exploitation of any discoveries. Further checks should be made at the various stages of patent filing. Analysis of patents can also give an indication of the competitor situation.

- Competitor information is important at all stages of the drug discovery and development process. Desktop databases can provide access to some of this information. Information professionals have a role in analysing and synthesizing competitor information from a wide range of literature, patent and drug pipeline databases to provide the complete competitor scenario.

■ Genomics/bioinformatics literature and databases. Here again the emerging role for the information professional is to work in closer partnership with the scientists. It requires a good foundation in these disciplines and in molecular biology, as well as the ability to help the scientists make the most effective use of the increasing range of databases and tools designed to access and analyse this information.

■ Internal/proprietary information is a significant component of the information managed within research information departments. Information professionals will be involved in the management and use of databases and services associated with internal records of biological, chemical, clinical and other R&D activities.

Some of the emerging challenges and opportunities in making optimum use of this information, and in dealing with the growth of information in this area are listed in Figure 10.4.

The issues/challenges faced by R&D and research information departments

Members of IMPI (Information Managers in the Pharmaceutical Industry) in the UK, of the PDR (Pharma Documentation Ring) in Europe, and of the DIA (Drug Information Association) in the USA are well aware of the challenges they face in the provision of information services, and often carry out benchmarks amongst themselves to determine best practice and how best to influence vendors in the industry. Jane Whittall, who is a member of the first two associations, has summarized some of the strategy and drivers for information provision (Whittall 1998):

■ increasing globalization of the pharmaceutical industry
■ knowledge management
■ need to demonstrate value and impact
■ new (information) technologies
■ the information marketplace
■ user behaviours
■ resources.

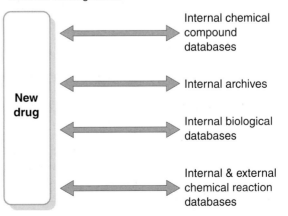

Figure 10.4 *New directions*

Related to these are also:

■ competitive pressures
■ increased cost of information (not just IT)
■ new R&D technologies creating new information demands.

Each item from the top list will be looked at in turn.

Increasing globalization

While many pharmaceutical companies now have operations in several countries, few are yet managing on a truly multinational basis. In 1998, only SmithKline Beecham was completely 'transnational' (i.e. with integrated US/UK organizations), although both GlaxoWellcome and Pfizer had managers responsible for multinational information resources, and other companies, such as Roche and the then Astra, had information departments which were beginning to operate transnationally. In a global environment, managers are more easily able to optimize the use of assets (e.g. employee expertise) and resources (e.g. library services, information and knowledge bases), and can also have more influence on information providers e.g. by negotiating global contracts. This must give them a competitive edge over other, more segmented, organizations.

Knowledge management

Knowledge management is described in more detail in Chapter 4. It is recognized as a major strategy for optimizing the competitive advantage of an organization. Both information departments and organizations as a whole need to identify ways in which they can:

■ enhance the use of their intellectual capital, e.g. in encouraging the sharing of knowledge
■ make optimum use of associated technology, e.g. by finding ways of recording expertise for wider use, but also by finding new ways of accessing the information already held in databases (data mining)
■ find ways to enhance the use of knowledge and expertise throughout the R&D process.

Value and impact

As already mentioned in this chapter, with the increased range of resources available to customers for obtaining their own information, information professionals have the opportunity, and indeed the responsibility, to focus on more value-added services, which will have a greater impact on the R&D process. Cost constraints and competitive pressures also provide impetus for this emphasis. We therefore need to identify key points in the R&D process where we can have a real impact, for example by providing the information and analyses which will support key decisions. We need to work in closer partnership with our customers so that we can understand and meet their needs, and also provide consultancy in the use of information resources.

New technologies: information and R&D

■ New information technologies include greater use of the internet and intranet, for access to external and internal information sources. The increasingly universal use of the worldwide web and its associated search engines provides information departments with the opportunity to provide an integrated front-end to the information resources, both databases and services, required by their customers. There are also increased opportunities for integrating both internal and external information sources to facilitate searching and decrease the need for familiarization with multiple front-ends. 'Push' technologies, which can deliver the latest information direct to customers' desktops can be both an advantage and a disadvantage. There is an indication of a trend back to 'pull' technologies whereby users can have more of an influence on what is actually delivered.

■ The new R&D technologies have already been mentioned earlier in this chapter. They too pose a challenge for information professionals, who not only need to familiarize themselves with the emerging disciplines, but will also need to revise the information processes and databases designed to manage this information. For example, new forms of chemical entities and larger volumes of data need to be handled by chemical registration processes and biological data systems.

The information marketplace

The information marketplace itself undergoes change on an ongoing basis. This continuously effects who we need to negotiate with, and the products and information strategies on offer. As pharmaceutical companies merge or change, we also have changing negotiation plaforms to work from, e.g. larger companies, more numerous sites, more global representation.

User behaviours

Influencing user behaviour is an ongoing 'challenge' for information professionals. Some of the changes which we experience may affect our users, and so have to be transmitted effectively. (See Chapter 15 for some of the ways in which we might effectively manage this change.) We need to recognize that different customer groups will behave differently in their preferences for types and designs of information products and services, but also need to influence them to make the most effective use of the new resources at their disposal. In SmithKline Beecham we found that whilst, as a rule, chemists are keen to use new information technology and carry out their own information searches, clinicians prefer paper-based information delivered to their desks and more personal contacts with information professionals. Again, Chapter 15 describes some of the different behaviours observed in the use of information resources.

Resources and cost saving

There are several trends and opportunities in these areas such as:

■ Cross-charging. Like all other departments, information departments will be subject to cost constraints. We need to develop models for how the provision of information resources is to be funded. Possibilities range from one end of the spectrum where the department bears all the cost, to the other where other R&D departments pay for their share of information sources and services.

■ Outsourcing. Again, there are a range of options available for using specialized external services or contract staff for carrying out such activities as abstracting, indexing, data input, literature searching.

■ Negotiation. As mentioned earlier, information departments need to find ways to negotiate the best deal with information providers or vendors through global licences which maximize the purchasing power of the company and through focus on licensing terms which confer advantage.

■ Benchmarking with the 'best in class', be they pharmaceutical or otherwise, provides insights into best practices and the best way of optimizing resources.

■ Information audits on the other hand will help departments identify what resources are being used throughout the organization, and hence may identify opportunities for better use of those resources. For example, where multiple subscriptions are being taken out with publishers there may be an opportunity to negotiate a common licence.

Chapter 11

Pharmaceutical commercial information

Ian Rowlands and David Bawden

Introduction

Pharmaceutical companies are commercial, as well as scientific entities, and produce and require commercial as well as scientific information. Indeed, the two aspects are impossible to distinguish clearly, in an environment where a share price may be dramatically affected by the leaked results of clinical trials, and where presentations of research concepts to financial analysts are at least as significant as those to scientific peers.

This chapter is therefore rather artificial, in apparently distinguishing one kind of information, and denoting it as 'business' or 'commercial'. It should be clear that the information content and resources described in other chapters of this book have a commercial significance.

The purpose of this chapter is to provide a forum for the description of the processes and sources important for the strictly business aspects of pharmaceutical information provision, and which are not mentioned elsewhere. It begins with an outline of businesses and business information per se, before concentrating on the two general topics of importance in this area: information on companies and information on the 'environment', including markets, competitors, and similar aspects.

The sources referred to, whether specifically geared to pharmaceuticals or more general in nature, are examples taken from the very wide variety available.

Information in business

Commercial organizations differ in many ways, and even a cursory examination of the business world reveals an enormous variety of business types: from the small local supplier of a single product or service to the multibillion dollar multinational corporation trading on a global scale. Regardless of size, method of financing, or sector, businesses share at least one common feature: their commercial activities are founded on their ability to source inputs from the external environment and to transform these into outputs which can be sold or traded. In fact all organizations, whether 'commercial' or otherwise, need to acquire a range of inputs (skilled labour, premises, technology, finance, materials) in order to be able to offer the goods and services (outputs) which their clients or paymaster demand (Fig. 11.1).

Even this simple input-output model of a business organization has some profound implications. If a business is to succeed, it must be able to identify suitable inputs and secure them at the lowest cost. It must be able to coordinate the use and deployment of these resources within the organization to maximum effect; and to add sufficient value to meet and preferably exceed the expectations of its customers.

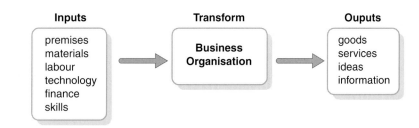

Figure 11.1 *The business organization as a transformation system*

An organization's need for resources makes it uncomfortably dependent upon the fortunes of the suppliers of those resources. Some features of the way that these resource markets operate can have a fundamental impact on the firm's success and on the way that it organizes its internal procedures and processes. By the same token, the success of suppliers is intimately bound up with the decisions and fortunes of their customers, as the decline of the UK clothing industry testifies. While a firm may decide to gain an advantage in price, quality or speed of delivery by switching to an overseas supplier, this in turn creates new uncertainties, not least potential fluctuations in currency exchange rates. Equally, firms may face uncertainty and change, even in domestic resource markets, as a result of technological change, government intervention or public opinion (as in the recent debate about genetically-modified foodstuffs).

Customers are vital to all organizations and the ability both to identify and to meet consumer needs is one of the keys to organizational survival and prosperity; a point not overlooked by politicians who are increasingly using business techniques to attract the support of the electorate. This idea of consumer sovereignty, where resources are allocated to produce outputs that satisfy customer demands, is a central tenet of the market economy and is part of an ideology whose influence has become all-pervasive in recent years. Understanding the many factors affecting both individual and market demand and the ways in which firms organize themselves to satisfy that demand is an essential element in surviving in a business environment that is increasingly market-led. In the pharmaceutical area, this is seen, for example, in the increasing pressure from health services for price controls, and in the increasing trends towards 'consumerism' among those taking the medicines which the industry provides.

Competition, both direct and indirect, is an important part of the context in which many firms operate and is a factor equally applicable to the input as well as the output side of business. The effects of competition, whether from domestic organizations or from overseas firms, is significant at the macro as well as the micro level and its influence can be seen in the changing structures of many advanced industrial economies. How firms respond to these competitive challenges and the attitudes of governments to anti-competitive practices is a legitimate area of concern for business information specialists. This has been put into sharp focus with the trend towards mergers producing 'mega-companies' in the pharmaceutical area.

Taking this systems approach, it is possible to reconceptualize the firm as an information system. None of the activities above is possible without adequate information. The firm must be able to turn as and when needed to the labour market to find managers, technologists, clerks; to the finance markets to raise capital or manage its cashflow; to the property markets to find suitable office or factory space. It must keep up to date with developments in management practice and thinking, like e-commerce or supply chain management, if it is not to be left behind by its competitors within the same industry, and it must always be one step ahead of its customers, sensing their emergent requirements perhaps even before they do so themselves. A pharmaceutical company must do all of these things, while also remaining entirely au fait with scientific and technical advances, and with changes in medical practice.

Table 11.1
Information in the life-cycle of a commercial product

Product life–cycle activity	Information need or activity
Generation of new product ideas	Brainstorming, possibly linking data from trade advertisements, competitors' catalogues, articles in the trade press
Screening new product ideas	Pitching ideas against the firm's mission, objectives and targets
Assessing market potential of new product	More brainstorming, linking data from consumer focus groups, published market research, demographic projections
Competitor analysis	Company annual reports and prospectuses, newspaper and trade press stories, patent filings
Research and development	Technical, environmental, legal and regulatory, patent information
Production	Production control (internally generated)
Distribution logistics	Distribution, warehousing, stock control, transportation, export duties and regulations
Product growth	Constant monitoring of sales, promotional efforts and the activities of competitors
Throughout the entire process	Management control, education and training

Adapted from Burke & Hall, *Navigating Business Information Sources*, 1998

Simply stated, business organizations are not closed systems. They operate in a complex web of overlapping markets, industry sectors and geographies in which access to inputs and the value of their outputs are hotly contested.

It is customary to distinguish between two general kinds of information which support the activities of a firm: internal information which is generated within the walls of the organization, often as a by-product of data systems which manage production, sales, payroll and invoicing processes; and external information which has to be sourced from outside, in the form of trade publications, online information services, commissioned market research or consultancy services. To some extent, this is an unnatural and unhelpful distinction since the primary value of information to a firm lies in its utility to the business rather than its point of origin. However, given that in most firms internal information is generally rather better understood and more fully integrated into its decision-making processes than most external information, the distinction is still useful in a diagnostic rather than a theoretical sense. Indeed, when one thinks of the nature of much external information—gossip about a forthcoming opportunity brought back from a medical symposium by the marketing team, a report on business conditions in Slovenia in the *Financial Times*, a profits warning issued by a major competitor, it is clear that very special skills of filtering and interpretation are needed.

The term 'business information', as commonly used, focuses on the external information needs of a firm and how such information can be integrated into more effective management decisions. To make this point a little more concrete, Table 11.1 relates business information needs and activities to the business processes involved in bringing a new product from the drawing board to the market.

Firms and industry sectors differ markedly in the intensity and breadth of their requirements for information at each of the stages above. Large, export-oriented firms in highly competitive markets will clearly require more depth in relation to competitor analysis and distribution logistics. Small, high technology 'Silicon Glen' companies will need to focus especially on idea generation and screening, while R&D-based pharmaceuticals companies will be acutely aware of the need for information to support their research and development activities. Burke & Hall's product life-cycle model reminds us that business information seeking is a highly directed activity, rooted in the needs of the business at various points in time.

From the material that has been presented so far, it will be clear that a succinct definition of what comprises 'business information' is going to be rather problematic. Michael Lowe defines business information as:

> ... *information on those factors outside and largely beyond the control of the business which may have a direct commercial significance. It is information on what has been called the external, or macro, or marketing environment, to distinguish it from a business's equally significant internal environment. Any factor in the external environment can be the subject of business information; but not everything about a factor has the direct commercial effect which distinguishes it as business information. External factors and the business information sources which report on them, fall naturally into 'domains'; it is common to refer to the major divisions of business information as 'company information'; 'market information'; 'City' or 'financial information'; 'product information'; and 'country' or 'geopolitical information'.*
> (Lowe, 1999: xviii)

This definition is valuable for two reasons: it is highly inclusive and it advocates a view of business information provision which emphasizes that it is, or at least should be, a highly proactive activity.

Competitive intelligence and environmental scanning

In many corporate environments, business information capture and analysis tend to take place on an ad hoc basis in reaction to external events such as the entry of a new player into the marketplace. Often the research brief is absurdly vague (typically 'finding out everything there is to know about...' the research target). The results of such projects tend to be highly speculative and often out of date by the time the project is complete. Furthermore, the concept of reacting to competitor initiatives is troublesome in terms of strategy and planning: the goal should be to anticipate. For this reason, many firms are beginning to appreciate the need for a more systematic and holistic approach to handling business information, making it an explicit activity within the context of strategic planning.

The term 'competitive intelligence' is sometimes used to describe the integration of business information activities with corporate strategy and planning. Competitive intelligence can support virtually any business function but obviously it is a fundamental component of strategy development and business planning, where it may be especially powerful. But competitive intelligence also supports tactical decision-making where it is typically applied with respect to discrete business functions. Some typical applications for competitive intelligence might include the following.

Mergers and acquisitions

In this area, of very clear significance in the pharmaceuticals arena in recent years, competitive intelligence is often used to contribute to due diligence in the investigations conducted after such plans are developed. However, providing more than the simple acquisition of historical financial data, competitive intelligence can help assess the future prospects for the merger candidate. In addition, it can be even more powerful in developing the understanding of competitors' capabilities, strengths, and weaknesses that could indicate a need for, or the desirability of, some type of business combination. Rather than limiting the horizon of a firm's merger activities to the relatively small pool of firms that are expressed or obvious candidates for an alliance, competitive intelligence can help identify potential partners in the larger pool of firms that are not obvious takeover candidates.

Marketing

Traditional market research is used to try to understand market preferences so that products which meet real needs can be developed. An understanding of a competitor's marketing strategy will not only help a firm to see how its competitors perceive the market (and confirm or negate its own perceptions), it may also indicate new areas of opportunity and vulnerabilities in its own plans. Knowing the market is important; but it is equally important to know where, how, and when competitors may attack. As a corollary, intelligence concerning a competitor's marketing plans, including what it does not intend to do, might save the firm from the expense of making pre-emptive moves in the wrong area.

Pricing and cost analysis

This is another area where competitive intelligence can play a vital role. Such knowledge is intimately related to strategic planning. Can the firm compete on cost, or should it attempt to differentiate its product in some other manner? Without knowledge of its competitors' cost structures and pricing policies, such decisions are made in a vacuum. But how is it possible to acquire such information? Cost and pricing data are among a firm's most closely guarded secrets (not to mention the charges of collusion that would occur if this information were shared). Obviously, some knowledge of the manufacturing and other business processes used is essential to such an assessment. Knowledge of the processes employed, the types and sources of raw materials used, and the distribution channels engaged will enable a firm to begin reconstructing a competitor's cost structure. Such knowledge is seldom available in a complete package but must be synthesized by the competitive intelligence analyst from numerous disparate fragments of evidence.

R&D and strategic technology planning

Building in large measure upon existing technology forecasting and data mining methodologies, competitive technology intelligence can provide needed background into technology trends and competitor capabilities and needs. New developments in scientometrics (including patent analysis, literature citation analysis), which rely on data mining techniques may provide additional insight into the technological landscape. In high-technology industries, such as pharmaceuticals, new discoveries appear at a rapid rate and patent monitoring is essential for those who want to stay knowledgeable. Patents are a unique source of competitive intelligence as well as technical information, and can be mined for insights into technology trends, revealing the commercial strategies and capabilities of rivals, and acquiring exclusive rights to emerging market-leading technologies.

All of these activities suggest the need for firms to be able to continuously monitor their external environment, not just react on an ad hoc basis. Environmental scanning is a widely accepted technique for monitoring the pulse of change in the external environment, whether it be in political, economic, technological, or social arenas. It can provide information to help guide institutional decision-making by alerting managers to trends and issues that may affect the organization's future. It is the process of identifying, collecting and analysing information pertinent to the organization's mission.

Environmental scanning involves regular, ongoing monitoring of direct competitors and their initiatives, so as to avoid surprises, as well as latent competitors (those who might become market entrants). However, environmental scanning does not necessarily turn up immediately useful nuggets of competitive intelligence. For example, a pharmaceuticals firm might learn that its main competitor has recently cited previous technologies in a patent application filed in Europe (patent applications are public documents in Europe, unlike the United States), while, at the same time, they have begun importing particular organic compounds from Brazil and have begun hiring scientists with expertise in a particular field of antibiotic drug approval. None of these pieces of competitor information means much on its own; it is the synthesis of the various bits of information that might lead the pharmaceuticals firm to begin drawing some conclusions about where its competitor is headed, perhaps foreshadowing the introduction of a new antibiotic compound some years in the future.

This is very much the nature of scanning one's competitive environment; bringing together the parts of an equation that represent meaningful advance warning of where a competitor might be headed in the future, rather than where it has already been. The firm that begins to integrate the workflow processes of ad hoc, event-driven research with those of environmental scanning begins to realize the true power of competitive intelligence.

Information about companies and investments

By nature, companies tend to be secretive, or at least highly selective, about the information that they release about their activities and performance to the outside world. And yet there exists a thriving and lucrative marketplace for company information products in the form of company directories, online information services, CD-ROM products and current awareness services. Dun & Bradstreet, Standard & Poor, Extel and Reuters all manage to run profitable publishing services in the company information area. How can this be?

Information about companies is made public in three major ways:

- voluntary disclosure
- disclosure by third parties
- statutory disclosure under company law.

Of course, voluntary disclosure is by its very nature haphazard and highly selective and may amount to little more than a corporate brochure, sales catalogue or website (although the latter form of disclosure is becoming an increasingly important business information resource).

In the course of discharging their responsibilities, businesses inevitably leave regular information trails with their suppliers, customers, banks and auditors. On a more infrequent basis, they will also be forced to disclose information to courts of law or to government agencies in respect of, for instance, levels of pollution emissions or a planned takeover or merger which might potentially result in the creation of a monopoly situation.

Potentially, such third party information disclosure, falling outside the provisions of company law, and certainly outside what might reasonably be expected of voluntary disclosure, may be a source of significant business intelligence (see Table 11.2).

While bankers and auditors require the client's permission before disclosing information, they may be able to supply references. In fact, much of the information in Table 11.2 is available to the public in the form of registry entries or reports, or may comprise data which can be sold on to information providers (information about payments, for instance, especially when involving credit).

For all that voluntary and third party disclosure are important weapons in the business information specialist's armoury, however, the information disclosed under the provisions of company law form the most widely consulted and structured company information resource. To understand the nature and extent of the information which businesses are obliged to make available through statutory disclosure, it is essential to have a basic understanding both of company law and the various ways that business units organize themselves and raise the finance they need to sustain and develop their activities. We shall see that there is a fine and delicate balance between a company's size, status and mode of financing itself,

Table 11.2 *Third party information disclosure*

Business transaction or relationship	Third party's knowledge
Buying	Payment record: size, speed, reliability
Selling	Capacity, quality, speed
Banking and auditing	Financial status, creditworthiness
Appearing in law courts	Transgressions, financial status, bankruptcies
Membership of stock or other exchanges	Detailed financial and operational data
Patenting a new invention	Detailed product or process information
Dealings with industry regulators	As above, plus details from enquiries
Compulsory notifications (e.g. emissions)	Details of chemicals and processes used
Government commissions (e.g. monopoly)	Details from enquiries and judgements

Adapted from Lowe, 1999

its ability to carry out its business in private, and the legitimate information needs of investors and regulators.

In the UK the simplest form of business organization is the sole trader. A sole trader is any private person who is engaged in business on his or her own account, someone who is, say, a self-employed builder or consultant. There are no information disclosure requirements other than those connected with income tax and (subject to turnover) with the payment of VAT and neither of these categories of information is in the public domain; this is entirely a private administrative matter between the sole trader and the state. Needless to say, such a situation is not likely to apply to a pharmaceutical company; though such companies, like any other, may need to deal with sole traders, and hence may need to find information about them.

The sole trader may operate his business under his own name, John Smith, or may assume a business name such as 'John's Reliable Motors'. In the latter case, John Smith would no longer be trading under his 'real' name and, in the UK, would be required to register the business name under the provisions of the Business Names Act 1985, which include a requirement to disclose ownership and an address at which notices can be served on all official business communications.

It is quite conceivable that John's second-hand car business becomes so successful that he needs to expand. He could employ extra staff to help out, or he might even decide to go into partnership with his main rival, Ron McNab. Ron would not only bring his expertise to the partnership but also an injection of cash and a share in future profits or losses. Legally speaking, a partnership is *'the relation which subsists between persons carrying on a business in common with a view to profit'*. In a general partnership, each partner is personally liable for the assets and obligations of the business, just like a sole trader, and the names of partners must appear on business documents such as the letterhead. Beyond this, only the business name, 'Smooth Runners', would need to be registered. John and Ron would still effectively be trading as private individuals and there would be no legitimate public interest in making their affairs more open to scrutiny, assuming that they were conducting their business affairs in an honest and professional manner.

The law generally discourages the formation of large partnerships (i.e. more than 20), with exceptions for professional firms such as solicitors, estate agents and consulting engineers which can grow to become very large international practices. Indeed, the presumption of the law is that for many sole traders and partnerships, further growth and expansion will come through incorporation and the possibilities for attracting new sources of financing that this opens up by the granting of limited liability status. The majority of larger traders opt to be private limited companies and to enjoy the privilege of limited liability.

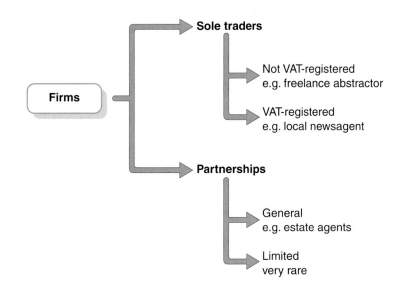

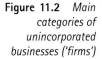

Figure 11.2 *Main categories of unincorporated businesses ('firms')*

As partners, John and Ron are fully responsible for any debts and liabilities that result from their second-hand car dealings. Potentially, this could mean losing their homes and savings and facing personal ruin. If, however, they formed a private limited company, 'Smooth Runners Ltd', their losses would be limited to the amount invested in the business. Importantly from a legal perspective, although the concept is perhaps rather difficult, a company has a legal personality in its own right which is independent of that of the owners. In other words, a company may enter into contracts and agreements, it may sue and be sued, and carry on regardless of changes of personnel. The legal penalties that can be imposed upon it are limited to fines, or in extreme cases, winding up.

Incorporation is a relatively easy process. Most solicitors will assist with the paperwork, or John and Ron could even buy a ready-formed company off-the-shelf by approaching a company formation agent. The vast majority of limited liability companies now registered in the UK are formed under company law and are registered with Companies House. There are a few exceptions to this rule: companies can still be created by Royal Charter or by Act of Parliament, but this is reserved for special cases and is no longer commercially important.

Incorporation and the privileges of limited liability bring with them a duty on the part of limited companies to make certain information about their activities public, indeed there is a statutory requirement for them to do so.

The Companies Registration Office (CRO), informally known as Companies House, is the state agency which is responsible for maintaining a register of UK limited companies and for ensuring that they comply with statutory requirements for information disclosure. These requirements vary depending on a number of factors, including size and legal status. Generally speaking, large private and public companies are required to make a great deal of information public, including details of their financial status and any information (such as changes of top personnel) which may affect the value of their shares. The requirements on small firms are much less stringent.

The central role of the CRO in the UK in corporate information gathering and dissemination cannot be overestimated (see Fig. 11.4). The CRO offers access to its corporate data at low cost and through a variety of routes: it is possible to consult its registers in one of its public reading rooms, obtain a fax or photocopy of a company's record by post or courier, or consult basic information online.

In line with prevailing government policy and an outlook which views some forms of information as a valuable commodity, the CRO also engages in licensing arrangements with

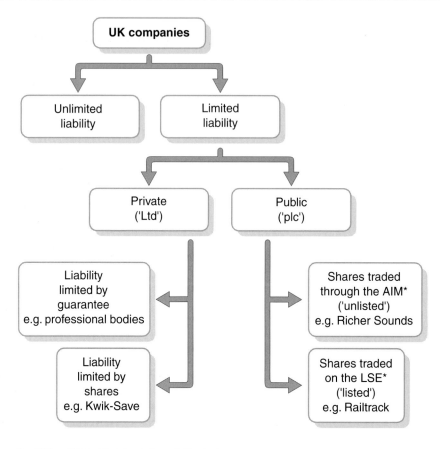

Figure 11.3 Main categories of incorporated businesses ('companies')

* AIM = Alternative Investment Market

* LSE = London Stock Exchange

'value-added resellers'—that is private sector organizations which take 'raw' CRO company records and add additional information of their own and provide for greater ease of access. Dun & Bradstreet, for example, enrich basic CRO records by including their own credit risk assessments, based on questionnaire returns and other in-house data, thus making the basic data more attuned to the needs of credit analysts. Dun & Bradstreet and other resellers may also make the basic CRO data more marketable by adding new search keys, like industry sector codes, which open up the possibility of drawing comparisons between companies more easily. The consumer thus has a choice between basic CRO data, whose collection costs have largely been met through the taxpayer, and more sophisticated information products and services with additional data and functionality which represent a commercial investment by private information industry.

On the basis of the CRO's willingness to enter into these commercial arrangements with value-added resellers, a large and complex marketplace now exists in the UK for the supply of extended information about companies. Space here does not allow for a detailed examination of the merits of the various sources; suffice it to say that choice, in terms of the data elements available, the way that these elements are organized and retrieved, and the delivery mechanisms (CD-ROM, paper, online, web) is enormous. Here the know-how of the business information professional is invaluable; first in decoding a client's real information need and then matching it with data from an appropriate source.

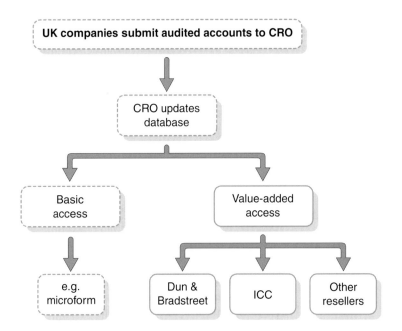

Figure 11.4 *Company information gathering and dissemination*

At the turn of the millennium, the corporate information sector is being shaken by the widespread availability of free information on the web and the subsequent devaluation of content. Content may no longer truly be king, but this only further emphasizes the importance attached to bundling and branding company information products effectively.

Nowhere is this statement more true than in relation to financial information, a term which is understood here as information on trading in financial instruments on national and international exchanges, rather than reports on a company's standing and performance as indicated above. The activities of 'the City' are at the very hub of commerce and power, and the financial services on offer to large companies enable them, among many others, to arrange financing, for growth or as part of a corporate restructuring package, to manage their cashflow, and to minimize the risks to their business associated with currency movements—particularly important of course for multinational businesses.

The information needed to support the workings of the financial markets obviously includes company information, in the rather limited sense outlined above. Indeed City institutions form the largest single market for company information products and services. However, this is only one element of the financial information environment, as anyone who has seen TV reports from a dealer's 'front office' will appreciate, with their images of traders surrounded by screens and telephones. The City may be a major consumer of historic company data, but its lifeblood is a continuous supply of instantaneous raw data: data concerning fluctuations in share values, prices of raw materials and currency movements which trigger buying and selling in financial instruments. In fact, so instantaneous are the information requirements that much trading is now triggered automatically by computer systems responding to certain price or index thresholds.

The real time data feeds which support trading mainly derive directly from individual exchanges such as the London Stock Exchange or NASDAQ, but they are supplemented by private sector information players (e.g. Bloomberg, Bridge, Dow Jones and Reuters) which add considerable value through extensive geographical coverage, historical depth, and the integration of financial data with news information. Dealers, and more particularly the analysts in the 'back office' who instruct them, must also monitor markets more widely. An

Table 12.2 *Strengths and weaknesses of spontaneous reporting systems*

Strengths	Weaknesses
Successful	Need substantive response within weeks
Data on exposure	Need data on exposure to New Chemical Entities
Useful for single drugs	Multiple drugs difficult
Useful for one outcome	Multiple outcomes difficult
Frequent events	Infrequent events
A mixed population	Specifically defined populations
–	Relative risk not yet possible
–	Risk for generic entities not possible
–	Risk for classes of drugs not easy
–	Long-term follow-up is not easy
–	Cause is not easy to assess

assessor reviews the information and reports back to a future meeting. Significant issues are entered onto a 'Business Activity' register to provide a tool for prioritizing, setting and monitoring targets for the further evaluation of signals. Note that the 'Business Activity' register may also be used to track signals in the literature, often reviewed as part of a separate process.

PSURs allow regular review of spontaneous reports. Guidelines for writing PSURs are detailed by the CIOMS II working group (CIOMS 1992). However, the European Committee for Proprietary Medicinal Products (CPMP) announced a change from CIOMS II to ICH PSUR in June 1997 (CPMP/ICH/288/95) and the MCA in the UK implemented the CPMP rules shortly afterwards. There are significant differences. Table 12.3 shows detailed differences between the data sets used in line listings for analysis.

The ICH PSUR requires unlisted rather than unexpected ADRs. This relates to the different information contained within PSURs around the world. Listed ADRs are in the core SPC. The core SPC contains mandatory information required in local SPCs although some regulators require additional information, including ADRs. It follows that the ICH PSUR requires a company to establish core SPCs. Thus, PSURs require analysis of the differences between local and core SPCs to ensure that information required by one country should not be included in the core. For guidelines on preparing core clinical safety information on drugs, see the CIOMS III report (CIOMS 1995).

The process of writing a PSUR (see 'Systems, processes and general principles', p. 173) requires support from the medical information department and collation of data not generally stored in pharmacovigilance such as exposure. Thus, medical information departments can play a key role in facilitating the PSUR process and other pharmacovigilance processes.

Post-authorization studies including pharmacoepidemiology are central to the future of drug safety. Epidemiology is the study of disease in defined populations. Pharma-

Table 12.3 *CIOMS II versus CPMP/ICH line listings*

Report Source	Selection for CIOMS	Selection ICH E2C
Spontaneous	All serious Non-serious unexpected	All serious Non-serious unlisted
Literature	As above	As above
Regulatory Authority	None	All serious
Consumer	Selected	If requested (separate)
Trials	Serious unexpected	All serious
Named patient	None	All serious

coepidemiology is epidemiological pharmacology. Abenhaim et al (1999) describe the relationship between pharmacovigilance and pharmacoepidemiology as ambiguous. For some people, pharmacovigilance includes all contributing methods including pharmacoepidemiology. For some, pharmacoepidemiology includes pharmacovigilance. Abenhaim et al distinguish between reporting-based systems identifying cases independent of investigator and epidemiological methods where case identification is investigator-driven. Venulet (1974, 1999) defined pharmacoepidemiology as '…science dealing with biological effects of pharmacologically active substances in populations exposed, regardless of reasons for such an exposure, which could be therapeutic or accidental or experimental or related to drug dependence'.

The importance of pharmacoepidemiology is illustrated by the formation of two new Divisions of Drug Risk Evaluation in the Office of Post-marketing Drug Risk Assessment at the FDA (Walker 1999). Based on pharmacoepidemiology, one of the highest priorities of the Office of Post-marketing Drug Risk Assessment is to explore the best way to customize post-marketing surveillance strategies for drugs reaching the market.

There are well established and described pharmacoepidemiological methods and databases that complement the activities of spontaneous reporting systems (McDonald 1994, Tilson 1998). Pharmacoepidemiology is about drug outcomes or outputs or events as numerator with the population at risk as denominator. The two main methods are case or cohort studies. A cohort-based approach in the UK is Prescription-event monitoring (PEM), linking prescriptions with adverse events of new medicines (Mann 1998). Automated record linkage systems and other developments in this area are well catalogued by the Risk Assessment, Detection And Response (RADAR) initiative. See section on 'Risk-Benefit', page 180.

Innovative approaches to risk and relative risk assessments using combinatorial approaches are developing. In pharmacoepidemiological analysis, linking information from governmental databases is growing. In the USA the FDA under Freedom of Information law makes the entire spontaneous AE database available to the public at nominal expense. There are many organizations that facilitate the obtaining of such information.

Selected data from the WHO Collaborating Centre for International Drug Monitoring, also known as the Uppsala Monitoring Centre (UMC), are available (UMC 1998). Although less complete than the information available from the FDA, that from the UMC is more international in scope, covering post-marketing reports supplied by various governmental health agencies to the WHO. It is most useful for data on products not yet marketed in the US. Beware of problems with taking these data out of context unless precautions are taken to ensure correct interpretation.

Literature

Despite its anecdotal nature and some poor documentation, literature remains one of the most useful sources of information on ADRs. Venning (1983) found that in discovering 18 important ADRs, the initial signal was through publication in almost all cases. Scanning journals, running routine online searches, using abstracting services and selective dissemination of information are all means of monitoring the literature for safety signals. There are many journals that publish relevant information on ADRs as well as specialist ADR-related journals (Talbot & West 1991).

The worldwide web is an increasingly useful medium for providing online access to bibliographic databases such as Medline. Other information on the web of relevance to pharmacovigilance includes:

- regulatory reporting guidelines by regulatory authorities
- associations dedicated to safety such as the Society of Pharmacoepidemiology
- ADR alerts such as 'Current Problems' by the MCA in the UK

■ press releases on safety issued by companies and news media
■ terminologies and networks relevant to safety.

Medico-legal aspects of pharmacovigilance

Under European Community rules, pharmacovigilance is one of several legal duties of the product marketing authorization holder. The broad legislative framework for licensing affecting pharmacovigilance consists of:

■ regulations—direct and immediate control
■ directives—require implementation
■ national law, e.g. product liability issues.

The current economics leads to more contracting in and out of services including pharmacovigilance. Whatever the contract, the product marketing authorization holder is responsible for pharmacovigilance. The consequences of failing legal duties include revocation or suspension of the licence with the following actions:

■ regulatory
■ criminal
■ civil.

Careful contractual drafting and pharmacovigilance procedures are essential. The following sections review issues about labelling in particular then medico-legal cases in general.

Labelling

Labelling in the context of pharmacovigilance refers to expectedness. Thus an expected ADR is a labelled ADR. Normally, changes are made to the labelling in the hope of controlling the risk-benefit ratio. Changes to labelling are triggered by:

■ direct request from the regulatory authority
■ requests from the company's pharmacovigilance department
■ signals from review such as PSUR or routine assessment
■ changes from mergers, acquisitions or process re-engineering
■ changes arising from local companies relating to core SPC issues—see 'Post-marketing', page 176.

Some repercussions to serious issues involving labelling changes can have similar effects as licence revocation. For example, the restricted use of desensitizing vaccines to centres with resuscitation equipment is described in the case history on desensitizing vaccines. Serious issues involving labelling changes include:

■ direct letters from the regulator or company to the doctor (Dear Doctor letter)
■ notification of problems through, for example, the MCA's 'Current Problems'
■ press releases about ADRs and risk-benefit
■ updates of related SPCs where ADRs are related to drug class effects
■ setting up of crisis or special project teams to deal with issues.

The process for updating SPCs generally has a large number of stakeholders. Communication between the stakeholders about these issues is a challenge particularly between headquarters, local companies and subsidiaries. Large changes may need ratification by directors although this level of authorization is avoidable. Smaller changes do not need agreement by all stakeholders. There may be resistance to updating SPCs. Thus 'freedom' to make such changes varies between companies. However, the actions taken by regulators may determine the overall changes. Labelling issues pose special problems in information and knowledge management.

Case study

1. In 1989, Current Problems published an article on anaphylaxis associated with desensitizing vaccines.
2. Data sheets were changed to allow only those centres with resuscitation equipment to administer the vaccines, leading to changes in marketing.
3. Use of vaccines fell.
4. A second Current Problems article was published in May 1994, 'Desensitizing vaccines: new advice'.
5. The overall effect over time of labelling changes in this case is more gradual than licence revocation.

Legal issues

Some of the regulatory consequences of legal issues are addressed in the labelling section. For a detailed review of the complex issues involving pharmacovigilance and regulatory actions, see Bendall (1998).

Civil issues generally relate to strict liability or to criteria for negligence. Strict liability came into force in the UK on 1 March 1988 with Part I of the Consumer Protection Act 1987, following EU Directive 85/374/EEC. Defective products are liable without the need to prove negligence. A product is defective when it does not provide the safety that a user is entitled to expect. The product must be shown to cause the injury suffered. The manufacturer of a product needs to be identified in a claim for strict liability or else the supplier may be held liable. Hospital pharmacists may be considered as suppliers if they formulate certain medications. It is interesting to note that hospital pharmacists are required to continue their insurance cover whereas pharmacists working within pharmaceutical companies are not. Very few cases involving the pharmaceutical industry and strict liability have been completely resolved.

Case study

To illustrate some of the issues for information management, a brief summary of the *Loveday* v. *Renton* case follows:

1. Susan Loveday, a 17-year-old with severe mental handicap, alleged that GP Renton was negligent in giving the combined vaccine including pertussis in 1970.
2. Wellcome's liability was not in question as the manufacturer was not known, however Wellcome conducted the defence.
3. An epidemiological study was used to show that the balance of probability was against pertussis vaccine causing brain damage.
4. The fact that there was no acceptable evidence that pertussis vaccine caused brain damage prevented further claims against Wellcome.

The criminal consequences vary from fines to imprisonment. Criminal sanctions for breach of pharmacovigilance requirements arise in the USA and several European countries. The EU has no powers of legal prosecution but does expect member states to enforce EU law with the same effectiveness as national law. Clearly, the implications for information and knowledge management are large.

Causality assessments

Stephens (1998b) wrote an excellent review of causality assessment. Causality assesses the likelihood that the suspected drug caused the AE in an individual case. The main aims of causality assessments are to satisfy legal reporting requirements and aid signal recognition.

However, there is not one clear methodology used by pharmacovigilance. Instead, there are at least 36 known methods, roughly classed into five types of assessment:

- global introspection, the differential clinical diagnosis similar to that used for any illness associated with a drug
- informal guides, such as Karch and Lasagna's method
- structural algorithms and decision trees, such as Hsu-Stoll method involving seven questions in an algorithmic format
- Bayesian logic, based on Bayes theorem for the relation that should exist between the probability of a population evaluated before and after the acquisition of new data
- expert systems, decision-making systems of which there are few examples at present.

For further detail of causality assessments and references, see Stephens (1998b). These five types of assessment refer to similar factors affecting causality including:

- the event
- time to onset
- dechallenge and rechallenge
- time to improvement or resolution
- reversibility
- dose relation
- different routes or dose
- concomitant medications and their indications.

The lack of reproducibility in methodology makes causality assessments a difficult field. Rather than evaluation and decisions made at the individual patient level, evaluation on behalf of the 'at risk' population from a public health perspective is central to risk-benefit.

Risk-benefit

The definitions for the purpose of this chapter are (Lawrence 1998):

- benefit is the probability that the patient benefits from the medication
- risk is the probability that something will happen.

Actual and perceived risks and benefits vary and risk is a topic in its own right, forming the foundation of the insurance business (Laudan 1994, Urquhart & Heilmann 1984). Over recent years, risk of Creutzfeldt Jakob association with bovine spongiform encephalopathy has not helped with perception of risk.

Evaluation

Lawrence (1998) summarized the evaluation of risk-benefit as follows: 'compare the interventions risk against the target-illness risk, weigh the benefits against the risks, and seek net risk reduction'. In general, the net risk-benefit profile for society must reflect how many patients are expected to benefit from a therapy and to what extent, along with the uncertainties. Although it is not possible to truly quantify a risk-benefit relationship, certain tools can strengthen the analysis and reduce weaknesses in judgement.

CIOMS Working Group IV (1998) is a good source of information on risk-benefit evaluation, with illustrative case histories in Appendix B. Risk-benefit methods can be descriptive and semiquantative or else quantitative. Descriptive methods evaluate benefits for a target disease as:

- seriousness
- chronicity
- extent of control or cure.

To exemplify a descriptive and semiquantitative method, Table 12.4 compares agranulocytosis occurring with dipyrone and gastrointestinal bleeding occurring with aspirin. Although the risks are similar, dipyrone was effectively removed from the Swedish and US markets in 1974 and 1977 respectively. In 1995 Sweden re-approved dipyrone for short-term treatment in specific groups of patients to obtain an acceptable risk-benefit ratio.

Quantitative methodology depends on the scales and weightings used. A method proposed by Amery (cited in Stephens 1998b) assigns risks and benefits scores that are combined into an overall therapeutic score. Different indications are associated with different risk-benefit balances. The goal is to place each drug in the risk-benefit spectrum by use of derived scores.

Actions to improve risk-benefit

CIOMS (1998) gives practical guidance to improve benefit-risk, with general principles including unresolved issues. Standard format and content of a risk-benefit evaluation report are recommended. The main outline is described here to show that addressing issues consistently for important safety issues of any type allows everyone to grasp the risks and benefits in a consistent way.

Introduction

Describe the purpose, inclusion of data from specified sources, included and excluded products. Specify the therapies selected for comparative analysis and your rationale. Consider advance agreement of the regulators on the selection.

Benefit evaluation

Describe the epidemiology and natural history of the target disease. Consider the purpose or intended outcome of the treatment, evidence for benefits along with alternative therapies.

Risk evaluation

Describe the general considerations in analysis including the specific ADR under analysis for preventability, predictability and reversibility. Identify the risk driver and effect on risk profiles then evaluate risk across products to obtain risk profiles for individual drugs, risk weighting and quantification.

Risk-benefit

Give the descriptive, semiquantitative or quantitative methods and analysis. Then summarize the general recommendations.

Table 12.4 *Dipyrone compared to aspirin (CIOMS 1998)*	Disease	Effectiveness of dipyrone	Dominant reaction	Disease	Effectiveness of aspirin	Dominant reaction
Seriousness	1	3	3	1	3	3
Duration	1	3	2	1	3	2
Incidence	3	0	1	3	0	2
Total	5	6	6	5	6	7

3 = high 2 = medium 1 = low 0 = no effect.

Options

Specify the options including monitoring, modification and decisions. Actions to improve risk-benefit and its assessment continue. Pharmacoepidemiological organizations along with proprietary pharmaceutical and disease outcomes research databases can assist with the risk-benefit analyses (see 'Post-authorization studies including pharmacoepidemiology', page 176).

Factors affecting drug safety

Genetics, pharmacokinetics and pharmacodynamics interrelate to affect the safety of drugs. Our increased knowledge of genetics and the human genome enables exciting discoveries in this area and is changing the face and future of clinical medicines and of pharmacovigilance.

Pharmacogenetics

Pharmacogenetics is the study of genetic variability and its effect on response to drug therapy. The key is linking computerized information about the nature, position and role of different genes in the disease process. Historically, genomics grew from Mendelian inheritance and was limited to looking for an unknown gene in people with a particular disease. Genetic variability in drug response was initially limited to measuring the responses to drugs and identifying differences at the level of genetic expression known as phenotypic, such as slow and fast 'acetylators' of specific drugs (Merck 1999). Now the genes of large populations are searched to see if known sequences of DNA are commoner in certain diseases (Bryan 1999). In the near future, our increased understanding will tailor the risk-benefit ratio to well-defined pharmacogenetic groups.

Developments in research and development methods include:

- collaborative research and sharing of information e.g. the Human Genome Project
- high throughput screening
- availability of very large databases for analysis in bioinformatics e.g. Genbank, SwissProt, Trembl
- large accessible populations.

These developments open the door to genetic profiling. A genetic profile is a tool for understanding an individual's susceptibility to medical disorders and how this may be addressed with new targeted drugs. Knowing a person's genotype may allow prediction of the risk of developing diseases. Genetic profiling has implications for preventive medicine, health insurance, employment, risks to offspring or siblings, ethical considerations. These factors come together in issues affecting pharmacovigilance such as patient identifiers allowing follow-up compared to data protection of the individual. Informed consent must be obtained from patients in genetics studies.

Pharmacogenetics has identified new diseases. One of the most important metabolizers of drugs is the cytochrome P-450 system (P450). P450 is involved in phase I metabolism of a wide range of drugs in liver cells. A variety of enzymes in the P450 system break down a wide range of drugs which compete with each other for metabolism via certain pathways. Also, some drugs act as inhibitors of P450 subtypes. For example, disulfiram inhibits subtype CYP2E1 while ethanol, isoniazide and paracetamol are substrates. Thus, pharmacogenetics has identified new diseases associated with different P450 subtypes and the journey to understand pharmacogenetics lies at this leading edge of research and development.

Drug metabolism etc.

In addition to pharmacogenetics, variations in drug responses are modulated by the following.

Pharmacodynamics and pharmacokinetics

One drug may alter the measured level of another drug by modulation at different sites to increase, decrease, multiply or add together its effects. Chronic or acute administration along with drug formulation affect kinetics and dynamics of the drug within the body. In turn, such effects are modulated by the following factors:

- drug metabolism and absorption are generally passive relating to formulation, pH and length of time the drug remains at the site of absorption. Change in extent of absorption results in variation in delivery of the drug to its site of action. Chelating agents and ion exchange resins can bind and decrease the extent of absorption. Malabsorption syndromes of folate, iron and vitamin B_{12} are caused by colchicine, neomycin and other drugs. Other substances such as grapefruit juice affect the absorption of drugs from the stomach
- distribution and excretion—most drugs are bound or actively transported in the body. Drugs inefficiently cleared by organs such as liver and kidneys are limited by binding. Displacement from plasma protein binding sites causes a rise in free drug levels. Moreover, permanent changes are seen in total plasma levels when total clearance of the drug is increased.

Given the complexity and interrelationship between drugs, ADRs and processes, it is interesting to see how far pharmacovigilance has come and to consider what the future may hold.

Good practice, the future and conclusions

Before concluding this chapter, it is appropriate to consider good practice in pharmacovigilance and briefly to look to the future.

Good practice

Good practice in pharmacovigilance does not yet exist compared to good clinical, manufacturing and laboratory practice. We do have key practices defined with recent publications including:

- CIOMS IV 'Benefit-Risk Balance for Marketed Drugs' (see page 180)
- Innovative development of risk and relative risk assessments (see page 181).

In addition, developments in neural networks and signalling may lead to improved practice in future. A signalling system using a neural network (Bayesian Confidence Propagation Neural Network) has been developed for mining data in the Uppsala Monitoring Centre database (UMC 1999). This tool uses Bayesian theory to quantify the degree to which a specific drug-ADR combination is different from a background, in this case the whole of the WHO database, and a confidence interval is calculated for each combination. By implementing the theory in a neural network, all drug-ADR associations in the database can be analysed quickly and automatically. Thus signals are highlighted on purely quantitative criteria. These highlighted associations can then be subjected to rigorous clinical assessment.

Pharmaceutical companies have to provide adequate resources in order to ensure compliance with regulatory guidelines for reporting. Paradoxically, this may be at the expense of good pharmacovigilance practice due to emphasis on meeting reporting requirements rather than resource improvement to risk-benefit of medicines. Enforcement of good clinical practice has made a difference to the standard of clinical practice. Thus development and enforcement of good practice in pharmacovigilance may improve product safety. However, factors such as political, social, economic and ethical issues impact pharmacovigilance in unpredictable ways.

The future

The future is driven by integration, convergence and linking resources together. Pharmacogenetics and pharmacoepidemiology are examples of the convergence of disciplines including genomics, epidemiology and pharmacology. The future of pharmacovigilance is in combining and collaborating between disciplines and stakeholders involved in the drug safety process. There are exciting developments in merging data with documents that may impact on pharmacovigilance in due course, such as shown by VHG™ (West and Murray-Rust 1999). The role of pharmaceutical information management underpins the success or otherwise of drug safety. Bringing information skills to pharmacovigilance functions requires deeper understanding of user needs and processes and vice versa. Future developments in integrating information and knowledge management should help, provided the fashionable trends are avoided and we continue to learn and manage the core information.

Conclusions

This chapter overviewed some of the aspects of regulations and guidelines affecting the reporting of ADRs. Although harmonization helps, there is a long way to go before regulators and industry work together collaboratively enough to improve pharmacovigilance measurably.

Managing information and knowledge is the key to the failure or success of drug safety. There is a revolution in communications such as the web, methodology, linking resources and pattern recognition that impact on knowledge (Bailey 1996). Thus there is an interesting future for pharmacovigilance.

References

Abenhaim L, Moore N, Begaud B 1999 Pharmacoepidemiology and drug safety 8: S1–S7

Bailey J 1996 After thought: the computer challenge to human intelligence. Harper Collins, New York

Begaud B 1993 Pharmacovigilance. Methodological approaches in pharmacoepidemiology. Elsevier ed ARME-P Bordeaux

Bendall C 1998 Legal aspects of pharmacovigilance. In: Detection of new adverse drug reactions. 4th edn. Macmillan, London ch. 14, pp 348–370

Bryan J 1999 Pharmacogenetics: choosing the best drug for the individual. Pharmaceutical Journal 262: 284–285

Council for the International Organization of Medical Sciences (CIOMS) 1990 International reporting of adverse drug reactions. WHO, Geneva

Council for the International Organization of Medical Sciences (CIOMS) 1992 International reporting of periodic drug safety update summaries. WHO, Geneva

Council for the International Organization of Medical Sciences (CIOMS) 1995 Guidelines for preparing core clinical safety information on drugs. WHO, Geneva

Council for the International Organization of Medical Sciences (CIOMS) 1998 Benefit risk balance for marketed drugs: evaluating safety signals. WHO, Geneva

Distillers Company 1961 Distival. Lancet 2: 1262

Food and Drug Administration (FDA) 1998 Federal code of regulations 21 CFR 312.32 IND safety reports, effective from 6 April,

FDA 1998 AERS http/www.fda.gov/cder/aers

Huntley C 1999 MedDRA has arrived: what should companies be doing about it? Good Clinical Practice Journal 6(2): 40–44

International Conference on Harmonization (ICH). April 1999 http/www.ifpma.org/ch1.html

Laudan L 1994 The book of risks: fascinating facts about the chances we take every day.

Lawrence Q 1998 Healthcare risks for health benefits. The Economist 19 September 50

Mann R 1998 Prescription-event monitoring – recent progress and future horizons. British Journal of Clinical Pharmacology 46: 195–201

McDonald R M and McDevitt D G 1994 The Tayside Medicines Monitoring Unit (MEMO). In: Strom B L (ed) Pharmacoepidemiology, 2nd edn. John Wiley, Chichester, pp 245–255

Merck 1999 Pharmacogenetics. Merck Manual http/www.merck.com/

Moride Y, Hurambura F, Requejo AA and Begaud B 1997 Under-reporting of adverse drug reactions in general practice. British Journal of Pharmacology 43: 177–181

Stephens M D B 1998a The methodology of the collection of adverse event data in clinical trials. In: Detection of new adverse drug reactions 4th edn. Macmillan, London, ch. 4, 97–129

Stephens M D B 1998b Casaulity assessment and signal recognition. In: Detection of new adverse drug reactions, 4th edn. Macmillan, London, ch.11, pp 297–318

Stokes T 1999 People, paper, and practices. How to survive the validation process and thrive on the business potential of strategic systems. Drug Information Journal 33: 49–61

Talbot J C C, West L J 1991 Sources. Drug Safety – shared responsibility, Glaxo Group Research. Churchill Livingstone, Edinburgh, ch. 11

Tilson H 1998 Pharmacoepidemiology in the pharmaceutical industry. In: Detection of new adverse drug reactions, 4th edn. Macmillan, London, ch. 8, 253–270

Uppsala Monitoring Centre (UMC) 1998 A network for safety: pursuing the optimal balance of risk to benefit for medicinal drugs worldwide.

Uppsala Monitoring Centre (UMC) 1999 Neural Networks http/www.who-umc.org/projects.html

Urquhart J, Heilmann K 1984 Risk watch: the odds of life. R R Donnelley, New York © Kinder Verlag, GmbH

Venning G R 1983 Identification of adverse reactions to new drugs. 2. How were 18 important adverse reactions discovered and with what delays? British Medical Journal 286: 289–292

Venulet J 1974 From experimental to social pharmacology Natural history of pharmacology. International Journal of Clinical Pharmacology 10: 203–205

Venulet J 1999 Epidemiological pharmacology. Pharmacoepidemiology and Drug Safety 8: 60

Waller P C, Coulson R A, Wood S M 1996 Regulatory pharmacovigilance in the UK: current principles and practice. Pharmacoepidemiology and Drug Safety 5: 363–375

Walker A M 1999 SCRIBE The International Society for Pharmacoepidemiology 2(2): 3,8

West L J, Murray-Rust P VHG™ 1999 http/www.vhg.org.uk

Further Reading

Benichou C 1994 Adverse drug reactions. A practical guide to diagnosis and management. John Wiley, New York

Council for the International Organization of Medical Sciences (CIOMS) Working Group I 1990 International reporting of adverse drug reactions. WHO, Geneva

Council for the International Organization of Medical Sciences (CIOMS) Working Group II 1992 International reporting of periodic drug-safety update summaries. WHO, Geneva

Council for the International Organization of Medical Sciences (CIOMS) Working Group III 1995 Guidelines for preparing core clinical-safety information on drugs. WHO, Geneva

Council for the International Organization of Medical Sciences (CIOMS) Working Group IV 1998 Benefit-risk balance for marketing drugs: evaluating safety signals. WHO, Geneva

Hartema A G, Porta M S, Tilson H H Pharmacoepidemiology 1999 An introduction, 3rd edn. Harvey Whitney Books, Cincinnati, Ohio

Lindquist M, Edwards R, Bate A, et al 1999 From analysis to alert—a revised approach to international signal analysis. Pharmacoepidemiology and Drug Safety 8(81):S15–S25

Stephens M D B, Talbot J C C, Routledge P A 1998 Detection of new adverse drug reactions, 4th edn. Macmillan Reference, London

Strom B L 1994 Pharmacoepidemiology 2nd edn. Churchill Livingstone, Edinburgh

Chapter 13

Regulatory affairs

Collette Beglin—Unicus Regulatory Services

Introduction

The pharmaceutical industry is perhaps the most regulated of all industries. Regulatory considerations affect all stages of the life-cycle of a medicine, not just the regulatory approval process itself. Pharmaceutical companies need to be fully aware of their regulatory responsibilities throughout a medicine's research and development programme, during the registration process, and thereafter when the medicine is on the market. This chapter explores the history of medicines control and describes the regulatory activities that pharmaceutical companies undertake.

The history of medicines control and regulatory affairs

Regulatory affairs is the mechanism by which a business deals with governmental controls and requirements specific to that business. The purpose of regulation is to protect the public in terms of restraining potentially incompetent or irresponsible industrial or commercial activities.

The history of medicines control can be traced back to ancient Greece and Egypt, where Galenic recipes for medicines were used. Later on, in the middle ages, Moslem medical practice involved standard methods of preparing medicines, and European craft guilds, peppers and apothecaries had their own recipes.

The 15th and 16th centuries saw the emergence of the first pharmacopoeias, including the London pharmacopoeia in 1618. The first British Pharmacopoeia was published in 1864.

By the late 19th century governmental regulations started to emerge, particularly in the USA. There was a crusade against patent medicines and quackery, which resulted in 1906 in the USA Pure Food and Drugs Act. This required labelling of named ingredients. It forbade the misbranding and adulteration of products and it forbade false or misleading promotion.

In the UK in 1925, the Therapeutic Substance Act was introduced. This covered the licensing of vaccines, sera, antitoxins and insulin.

In 1937, sulfanilamide elixir was marketed in the USA. It was labelled 'elixir' but contained diethylene glycol rather than ethanol. It caused 107 deaths, which were mainly in children, and was withdrawn under the Pure Food and Drugs Act for misbranding. This was an important case because it brought about the 1938 US Food, Drug and Cosmetic Act which, for the first time, saw the introduction of safety (in addition to quality) as a criterion in regulatory controls. This Act required prior approval of new drugs before they could be commercialized.

The third element of regulatory control, efficacy, was introduced following the thalidomide tragedy. In 1957, thalidomide was marketed in Germany for anxiety, insomnia, emesis and various other dubious indications. In 1958–59 it was also marketed in the UK, other European countries, Australia and Canada. It was widely prescribed for morning sickness but in Canada was only approved for anxiety and insomnia. In 1960, thalidomide was submitted for approval in the USA. Francis O'Kelsey, the assessor at the Food and Drug Administration (FDA), queried the peripheral neuropathic symptoms reported since the product had been marketed elsewhere. The same year, German paediatricians identified a new congenital deformation, phocomelia, or sealed limbs. In 1961 there was a rapid increase in cases of phocomelia, not only in Germany but also in other countries, particularly Australia. In November 1961, the German authorities announced a suspected link between the drug and phocomelia. As a result thalidomide was withdrawn from most markets and it was rejected in the USA. Canada delayed the withdrawal until March 1962.

The thalidomide disaster was a very significant event in the history of medicines control. It resulted in the USA, in 1962, in the Kefauver Harris amendments to the Food, Drug and Cosmetic Act. This gave virtual carte blanche to the FDA. It established efficacy as a criterion for approval. It required prior approval for new investigational drugs and it established the requirements for good manufacturing practices (GMP).

In the UK at the same time, 1962, the UK Dunlop Committee was formed. This was the forerunner of the Committee on Safety of Medicines which still exists today.

The three criteria for medicines control, quality, safety and efficacy, were adopted by countries around the world. During the late 1960s and 1970s the demands on pharmaceutical companies in terms of regulatory requirements increased immensely. There were also great variations in international regulatory requirements, which resulted in an increasing need for multiple studies, if not entire development programmes, in order to get just one product onto the market. This lengthened the drug approval process to an average of 12 years and also meant huge increases in the drug development costs.

Significant amendments to regulatory controls were brought about in 1983 with the US Orphan Drug Act, which provided incentives to manufacturers to develop drugs for rare disorders. In addition, in 1984, the AIDS epidemic saw the emergence of patient activism, with political pressure on regulators to facilitate the development of new drugs. Between 1985 and 1987, revisions to the procedures for New Drug Applications (NDA), and Investigational New Drugs (IND), were put in place. The US FDA reformed its drug approval process to encourage new drug development.

Between 1965 and 1990, the European Union went through a phase of major development. Of particular relevance for the pharmaceutical industry were harmonization of regulatory standards and requirements among individual member states and completion of the common European market. As a result of the attempt to harmonize in Europe, regulators and the pharmaceutical industry started to ask the question: 'If we can harmonize in Europe, why not globally?'

Then, in 1990, the International Conference on Harmonization was instituted. This was an effort between the European Union, the USA and Japan to consider common guidelines for drug development and registration in the three regions.

The rationale for new regulatory harmonization covers a number of key points. They include: the standardization of basic technical requirements; the identification and promotion of best practices; the free movement of goods in commerce; the portability of goods by travellers; minimization of development costs and minimization of consumption of test animals.

Recent developments in the history of medicines control include new registration procedures in the European Union, namely the centralized procedure and the mutual recognition procedure. There has been increasing recognition of EU standards and, in some cases, European approval outside the European Union. All of the harmonization initiatives around the world have meant shortening of drug development times and globalization of development programmes.

Legal framework of regulatory controls

Regulatory requirements are made up of laws, guidelines and ad hoc regulatory advice. Laws are of course legally binding requirements. They must be complied with and the regulators must enforce them. Legislation is usually difficult and slow to enact or amend. It is normally quite general leaving the regulators scope for interpretation. The UK Medicines Act and the US Food, Drug and Cosmetic Act are basic public laws concerning medicines.

Guidelines are not legally binding requirements. They are interpretations by the regulators of legally binding requirements and should normally be complied with. In certain circumstances, however, it may be justifiable to deviate from guidelines. They may be enforced by the regulators in a measured fashion, on a case-by-case basis. They are normally easy to promulgate and revise.

The other type of regulatory requirement is ad hoc regulatory advice. This is non-binding advice on a subject-by-subject or product-by-product basis.

European Union legislative instruments include directives, regulations and decisions. Directives are instructions to member states to approximate national laws. Regulations are legally binding on the entire European Union. Decisions, on the other hand, are legally binding specifically on those to whom they are addressed.

The International Conference on Harmonization (ICH) has representatives of the pharmaceutical industry from around the world and governmental regulators from Europe, the USA and Japan. In addition, there are a number of observers from the World Health Organization, the European Free Trade Area, and Canada. The ICH has a steering committee, with representatives from each of the main players plus the observers. There are also four expert working groups covering safety, quality, efficacy and multidiscipline topics.

The ICH process includes five steps:

- Step 1: the preparation of the first draft of a guideline for the steering committee.
- Step 2: the release of the draft guideline by the steering committee for external comment.
- Step 3: the revision of the draft guideline on the basis of the external comments received.
- Step 4: the approval by the steering committee of the draft guideline and its recommendation for the adoption in the three regions.
- Step 5: the incorporation of the guideline into the appropriate administrative measures by the various regions represented by ICH.

There have been a number of successes and failures in the ICH process. They relate to whether a consensus has been agreed on the original divergent requirements between the three regions, or whether a summation of the three regional differences in legislation has occurred. Consensus means the reconciliation of divergent requirements through compromise. This leads to a reduction in the multiplication of studies and agreement on study design and data requirements that reduces the total amount of work required for a global development project. Summation of differences, on the other hand, means the reconciliation of divergent requirements through the adoption of everybody's requirements, with little or no reduction in multiplication of studies. This type of agreement fails to reduce the total amount of work required for a global development project.

These issues may be illustrated by considering the output of the expert working groups on quality, safety and efficacy. Many examples of consensus on quality matters have been achieved. An example is the agreement on storage conditions for stability studies. In the area of safety there are also many examples where consensus has been achieved. Examples are the agreement on common toxicological protocols, the choice of animal species, etc. However, in the area of efficacy there are many examples of summation. The common clinical trial report guidelines, for example, incorporate the requirements of all the three regions.

Harmonization of legal and other instruments of medicines control will continue in the future. In addition, the process for updating and supplementing the current ICH guidelines will be put in place. Use of the ICH guidelines will be monitored and collaboration and exchange of information on newly emerging issues will help foster harmonization.

Regulatory agencies: structure and responsibilities

Most countries around the world have their own national regulatory agency or authority. Each authority is responsible for regulating the supply and sale of medicinal products in its country. In the UK, the regulatory authority is the Medicines Control Agency (MCA), which is located in London. The European Agency for the Evaluation of Medicinal Products (EMEA), is also located in London. The two agencies have very different roles.

The MCA has five separate business units. These comprise Licensing, Post-Licensing, Inspection and Enforcement, Executive Support and Finance. The MCA has a staff of over 400. Information about the roles and activities of each unit can be found at the MCA website (www.open.gov.uk/mca/homemain.htm). For the purposes of this chapter, only the Licensing and Post-Licensing divisions will be considered further.

The Licensing division of the MCA is responsible for the assessment of all new marketing applications and clinical trial applications in the UK. In addition, it has responsibility for the British Pharmacopoeia. The division is split into five groups. One deals with licensing applications for new chemical entities. Another handles abridged licensing applications for well-established active ingredients. A third deals with licensing of biological and biotechnology products. A fourth group handles clinical trial applications. The final group is responsible for the British Pharmacopoeia.

The Post-Licensing division of the MCA has a number of functions. It is responsible for pharmacovigilance and runs the UK spontaneous adverse drug reaction reporting scheme (the 'yellow card' system). It is responsible for variations and renewals of marketing authorizations. It also deals with changes in classification, for example if a company wishes to reclassify a product from 'Prescription Only Medicine' (POM) to 'Pharmacy' product (P), so that it can be bought at pharmacies without a prescription. The Post-Licensing division also has responsibility for regulation of product information (e.g. summaries of product charactersitics and patient information leaflets) and of advertising and promotion of medicines.

The MCA has as an expert advisory committee, the Committee on Safety of Medicines, the CSM. This committee advises on safety, quality and efficacy issues for new drugs. It also monitors all drugs on the market by the review of adverse drug reaction data and gives advice on licensing requirements.

The Medicines Control Agency has as its objective the role of protecting the patient population of the UK. It does this by controlling quality, safety and efficacy of all medicinal products on sale on the UK market and regulating companies that intend to apply for licences or conduct clinical trials.

The European agency, the EMEA, has as its objective the promotion of public health and the free circulation of pharmaceuticals in the European Union. The EMEA is split into three distinct functions: the management board, the scientific committees and the secretariat.

The management board is the supervisory body responsible for budgetary matters. It is comprised of representatives from each member state, from the European Commission and from the European Parliament.

The EMEA has two scientific committees: the Committee for Proprietary Medicinal Products (CPMP) and the Committee for Veterinary Medicinal Products (CVMP). Both committees meet every month and have 30 members, with two from each member state. The members are appointed because of their experience in medicinal product evaluation. The role of the committees is to give independent scientific advice to the EMEA.

The secretariat provides technical and logistical support. It is responsible for project management for products being assessed for marketing in Europe as a whole.

In the United States of America the regulatory authority is the Food and Drug Administration (FDA). The objective of the FDA is to protect the health and safety of consumers by ensuring that drug, biological and medical device products are safe and effective, and by ensuring that foods and cosmetics are safe and are made under sanitary conditions. The head of the FDA is a political appointee as part of the US government.

Within the FDA the Center for Drug Evaluation and Research (CDER) assesses drug applications for their suitability for the USA market. All staff of the CDER are employees and not political appointees. The FDA employs around 2000 staff. They are mostly based in Washington but there are also regional offices around the country. Typically these regional offices are charged with such things as inspection of good laboratory practice (GLP), good clinical practice (GCP) and food inspection. The FDA is responsible for all drugs including ethical, generic, over-the-counter (OTC) and veterinary medicines, and for most food except meat and milk, which are covered by other agencies. It is also responsible for medical devices, all biological products, and foods and cosmetics.

The CDER is split into groups responsible for particular therapeutic areas. For example, one group deals with gastrointestinal drugs and another deals with anti-infectives and antivirals. The members of these groups are specialists in their particular areas.

Role and activities of regulatory affairs departments in the pharmaceutical industry

There is no typical regulatory department. Regulatory departments are structured very much to meet the specific business needs of their companies. However, there are some common aspects. In particular, all regulatory departments are responsible for the registration of new medicinal products, including those used in clinical trials, and for the maintenance of existing marketing authorizations or product licences.

Regulatory departments are responsible for tailoring data generated during research to the needs of the regulatory authorities for each market in which the company is involved. The ultimate aim is to gain marketing approval of the company's products in the quickest way possible. Regulatory departments provide input at all stages of research and development. They may advise on the type of data that should be generated and on the studies that should be done to achieve the quickest approval in all the countries in which the company wishes to market the product.

The regulatory department plays a key role in ensuring that the marketing authorization is kept up to date at all times. Most regulatory authorities require the submission of a renewal application for every product on the market every five years. The regulatory department is responsible for filing this renewal in a timely manner. In addition, there may be changes to products' formulations, doses, side-effects, manufacturing methods etc. It is the responsibility of the regulatory department to ensure that all such changes are communicated to the regulatory authority and that approval is obtained through variations to the marketing authorization before the changes are implemented.

Registration has come about to ensure the safety of the patient by controlling the quality, safety and efficacy of all medicinal products on the market. It is there to protect patients from false medical claims, to control the dose of the product, to control purity and to prevent incorrect use of drugs.

As discussed at the beginning of the chapter, regulatory controls in some form or another have existed for many hundreds of years, but it was only during the 20th century that the controls as we know them today were formulated. In the UK, as a result of the thalidomide tragedy, the Medicines Act was introduced in October 1968. This granted all products that were already on the market a 'product of licence of right', but put in place a programme for reviewing all the data for all products. By 1991 all products on the UK market had been assessed by the regulatory authority. In addition to this, in 1971, product licensing became mandatory and all new medicinal products entering clinical trials or proposed for marketing had to be assessed by the licensing authority for quality, safety and efficacy.

There are a number of regulatory controls to govern the pharmaceutical products entering the UK market. The first is the product licence or marketing authorization. This must be held by the company or person responsible for the composition of the product or for placing the product on the UK market. The manufacturer of any product on sale in the UK must also hold a manufacturer's licence. This is only granted once the Inspection and Enforcement Division of the MCA has inspected the applicable manufacturing plant to ensure that it has the appropriate facilities and expertise to carry out the relevant process competently. The manufacturer must, of course, comply with standards of good manufacturing practice (GMP). In addition to these controls, all wholesale dealers must hold a licence. Similar to the manufacturer's licence, the wholesale dealer's licence is given by the Inspection and Enforcement Division when it is satisfied that the wholesaler has competent staff, procedures and facilities on site. A further method of control is that the Inspection and Enforcement Division is empowered to purchase samples of products from retail outlets and submit these for analysis. Where a defective product is released for sale or a product deteriorates abnormally a company is expected to have a batch recall system in place to ensure that the product can be withdrawn from the marketplace in a timely manner.

Regulatory activities during product development

During product development the role of the regulatory professional is to ensure that the project team works towards a regulatory strategy. This should identify the countries where clinical trials will be carried out, the registration route for the product in Europe, and the markets outside Europe that will also register the product.

Each phase of clinical development requires an application to be submitted to the regulatory authority. The exceptions are phase I studies in healthy volunteers, which in the UK do not require a clinical trial application to the MCA.

The submission to the regulatory authority at each phase of the clinical trial programme includes up-to-date pharmacy information, results from the ongoing animal work and any clinical information obtained. Thus at each phase of clinical development the dossier on the product grows.

Phase I of clinical development is usually the first approach to a regulatory authority. This is when the compound is first administered to man—to healthy volunteers rather than patients. Phase I studies are small, usually involving 20–80 subjects. They provide the initial clinical work which, together with the animal studies, will provide the basis for moving into phase II.

Phase II concerns the first administration of the compound to patients. Phase II studies are fairly small, typically involving between 100 and 200 patients. The aim is to find preliminary evidence about the efficacy of the compound and about its safety.

The bulk of the clinical development programme occurs in phase III. Here the objective is to confirm the dose that will be marketed, to establish the efficacy in specific indications, and to investigate use in specific patient populations. Often, during initial development of the compound, specific populations are chosen rather than including all possible patient groups. In Europe phase III may involve comparative studies against the products already on the market. It is also the phase in which the product's safety profile becomes more clearly defined.

In the USA there is a different approach to phase III clinical trials. Instead of comparative studies, the company is required to carry out placebo-controlled trials.

To satisfy all the regulatory authorities around the world, when companies put together a development plan they often put in place a three-arm study. Patients are treated with the new compound, the comparator product or placebo. Typically a phase III study covers between 1000 and 3000 patients.

During drug development the regulatory department should be working with the various groups within the company to decide when final study reports should be written and who will write them. The regulatory department may write the reports or they may be written by the research and development groups that have carried out the studies.

An important aspect of regulatory work during product development is to keep abreast of current legislation in the markets in which the company intends to register the product.

The company needs to be aware of any new legislation which may come into force by the time the company launches the product and which may affect the assessment of the application by the regulatory authorities.

Marketing authorization

A registration dossier in Europe is called a marketing authorization application. The structure of the dossier can be the same, regardless of whether it is submitted to one country for national approval or through the harmonized procedures for Europe-wide approval. The marketing authorization application, or MAA as it is known, is made up of four parts. Part I is a summary of the dossier, part II is the chemical, pharmaceutical and biological documentation, part III is the pharmaco-toxicological documentation, and part IV is the clinical documentation.

Part I of the dossier is made up of:

- an application form
- the summary of product characteristics
- any summary of product characteristics already approved in other European Union states
- the proposals for packaging, labelling and the pack insert
- the expert reports, perhaps the most crucial part of the whole of the MAA.

There are three expert reports, one on the chemical, pharmaceutical and biological documentation, one on the toxicological and pharmacological documentation, and one on the clinical documentation. These expert reports are written by either internal or external experts, who are chosen by virtue of their expertise and experience within the pharmaceutical industry. The expert reports are not a summary of the dossier. They provide analyses of the most important findings about the product from the research and development programme and the reasons why the company considers that the product should be granted a marketing authorization.

Part II of the dossier discusses the composition of the product, in other words how the particular ingredients were chosen and how the quantities of those ingredients were decided. It provides information on the method of preparation of the product and the quality controls used for the starting materials and the finished product. It also provides details of the container. Stability data for the active substance and the finished product are included, providing evidence that the product is stable for the proposed shelf-life.

Part III concerns the pharmaco-toxicological documentation. It gives the findings from single-dose and repeat-dose toxicity studies in animals and tests on the reproductive function of the animal species chosen. It includes information about embryo-fetal and perinatal toxicity as well as mutagenic and carcinogenic potential. Part III also provides details of the drug's pharmacodynamics and pharmacokinetics in animals.

Part IV concerns clinical pharmacology. It covers the product's pharmacodynamics and pharmacokinetics in humans and the clinical experience to date. The clinical dossier should be based on the proof of concept theory, in other words all products are assumed to be ineffective and not safe until proved otherwise. It is the responsibility of the company to prove the claims for efficacy and safety beyond reasonable doubt.

In 1995 the free movement of medicinal products in the European Union, comprising 15 member states and 370 million citizens, became a reality. At the time of writing, the member states of the EU are Austria, Belgium, Denmark, Finland, France, Germany, Greece, Ireland, Italy, Luxembourg, the Netherlands, Portugal, Spain, Sweden and the UK. All other European countries follow their national regulatory procedures.

When a pharmaceutical company is developing a new medicine, or a new formulation or line extension of an established product, it has to make a decision on how to file the marketing authorization application in Europe. There are three choices. If the company intends to register and sell the product in only one member state, it is still possible to file a national marketing authorization application. If it intends to market the product in more than one member state it must choose either the centralized registration process or the mutual recognition procedure.

The centralized procedure

The centralized procedure is compulsory for medicinal products derived from biotechnology. It is also available on request for highly novel new products. Using this procedure, the applicant makes a marketing authorization application submission directly to the EMEA in London. Scientific evaluation is then undertaken within 210 days. The Committee for Proprietary Medicinal Products (CPMP) provides its opinion and within a further 90 days the opinion is transformed into a final decision. If the opinion is positive a single authorization applying to the whole of the EU will be granted.

Details of the procedure

Once a company has submitted a dossier to the EMEA, it is checked for completion (the 'check-in' process). The EMEA selects a rapporteur, the national regulatory authority of one of the member states, to carry out the assessment of the dossier on behalf of the EMEA. The role of the rapporteur is to ensure good coordination between the EMEA, the CPMP and the company involved with the MAA. Day 1 of the evaluation is the day on which the CPMP receives the valid application after it has been through its check-in procedure and the rapporteur and co-rapporteur, if appropriate, have been nominated. The secretariat of the EMEA informs the applicant of the rapporteur and the timetable for the assessment of the application.

By day 90 the rapporteur must circulate a preliminary assessment report to the CPMP. The CPMP has until day 120 to consider this report and to establish which issues the applicant will be invited to clarify. At this point the clock stops since the applicant is asked to prepare written responses to a list of questions raised by the rapporteur and the CPMP. The clock only restarts when the applicant submits written responses to all questions. By day 150 the rapporteur prepares a report with the conclusions on the written responses of the applicant and circulates this to the applicant and to the CPMP. By day 180 the CPMP and the rapporteur must have discussed the findings and the written responses and must have decided whether to invite the pharmaceutical company to an oral presentation to explain any issues that are still not clarified. Finally, by day 210, the members of the CPMP must conclude the evaluation and adopt an opinion. If the opinion is positive a single European marketing authorization will be issued within 90 days and the company can launch the product in the European Union.

The mutual recognition procedure

The mutual recognition (MR) or decentralized procedure is applicable to the majority of conventional (non-biotechnology) products. The MR procedure is based on the principal of mutual recognition among member states of the assessment and approval made by one member state's regulatory authority.

Details of the procedure

The pharmaceutical company first chooses the EU member state whose regulatory authority it wishes to approach (the reference member state or RMS). It makes its MAA submission to that authority, which then carries out the assessment on behalf of Europe. The RMS has a total of 210 days to assess the application and, if appropriate, to issue the first authorization. During the 210–day assessment period the company is required to clarify and answer questions that the RMS raises. Once the RMS has finished its assessment it has a total of 90 days in which it must issue an assessment report. At the same time the pharmaceutical company must update the initial dossier to deal with all of the questions raised. At the end of this 90–day period, when the assessment report and the updated dossier have been completed, the applicant can request mutual recognition of the first authorization by the other member states. The company can choose one or more or all of the other member states (known as concerned member states or CMSs) in which to have the opinion of the RMS recognized. The CMSs have a total of 90 days to decide on mutual recognition of the authorization. If they have any queries or require further clarification these must be addressed to the applicant within the first 60 days of the 90–day period. After the 90 days, if there are no further issues and the CMSs have agreed on a decision, the marketing authorizations will be approved. The company then receives up to 15 harmonized national marketing authorizations.

Regulatory activities after registration

Pharmacovigilance

When a company receives a marketing authorization for a medicinal product, it must continue to satisfy regulatory and marketing requirements. In particular, effective pharmacovigilance systems must be in place to ensure the collection of all safety data and adverse event reports relating to the product.

There are of course many sources in which new information about a product may appear. Companies scour journals, letters, case reports, study reports, investigational reports and monitor ongoing clinical work for new information on their medicinal products. Adverse event information will also be received through spontaneous reports from physicians, pharmacists and sometimes directly from patients.

Companies have a responsibility to gather pharmacovigilance information and to report it to the regulatory authorities. Depending on the medicinal product and on the severity of the adverse event, there are different reporting requirements. For new chemical entities all suspected reactions should be reported to the regulatory authority, whereas for established products serious or unexpected reactions must be reported. Serious events are defined as life-threatening, fatal, incapacitating or requiring prolonged hospitalization. Typically, a serious adverse event must be reported to the appropriate regulatory authority in a matter of hours, whereas details of non-serious adverse events can be submitted in regular reports.

In the UK the Committee on Safety of Medicines, which is part of the MCA, has responsibility for reviewing adverse event reports. If it identifies significant changes to the safety profile of a product it can direct the pharmaceutical company that markets the product to make changes to the summary of product characteristics. If severe side-effects are identified it can, if necessary, order withdrawal of the product from the market.

Changes to the marketing authorization

In Europe a marketing authorization for a medicinal product is granted for a period of five years. It may be renewed at the end of this time upon application.

A company may also wish to make changes to a marketing authorization. Experience with a product after it has been approved generates much new information. Adverse events or drug interactions may be detected that did not occur in clinical trials. Further experience in clinical trials may lead to new indications. As a result the prescribing information during the first few years of marketing may need to be updated periodically. These updates require changes to the marketing authorization, which can be filed with the regulatory authorities as variations. Within Europe there are three types of variation: type I, type II and safety restriction.

Type I variations

An example of a type I variation would be a change in name of the product, either the trade name or the common name. As long as the proposed name is distinct from that of any other product on the market and is not likely to cause confusion, such a change is likely to be approved as a type I variation.

In general the information presented for a type I variation includes revised drafts of the summary of product characteristics, the patient information leaflet and labelling, and adequate justification for the change, plus any other relevant documentation. After the submission has been made the regulatory authority has 30 days to make a decision.

Type II variations

More substantial changes to the marketing authorization are covered by type II variations. As with type I, the company should submit revised drafts of the summary of product characteristics, the patient information leaflet and labelling, with documentation to support the proposed change. The regulatory authority has 90 days to make a decision.

Safety restriction

The third type of variation is an urgent safety restriction. This is an interim change by the authorization holder which has a bearing on the safe use of the product. For example, it may be necessary to restrict the indication and/or the dosage of the product, or to add a contraindication or a warning. In such a case the marketing authorization holder informs the regulatory authority and if no objections are raised within 24 hours the urgent safety restriction may be introduced. The corresponding application for a variation to the marketing authorization must then be submitted without delay.

Change to over-the-counter use

A company may decide to switch a product from prescription-only status to over-the-counter (OTC) use. To do this the company must have gathered sufficient safety data to ensure that the product will be safe for this wider patient use. A condition for approval of a switch to OTC use is that the indication must be easy for the patient to diagnose. The dose may be lower than is the case for the prescription product. Any change to the indication or dose will require further clinical studies. If, however, the OTC formulation is used for the same indication and at the same dose as the prescription product, the clinical dossier is based on the experience gained with the prescription use of the product.

Generic product registration

Once the patent on a medicinal product expires, it is possible for other manufacturers to produce generic versions containing the same active ingredients as the original. To register a generic product, the manufacturer can submit an abridged marketing authorization application. Before beginning development work, however, the applicant must ensure that the originator ingredient and product patents have expired and that the product has been on the market for a number of years within the European Union.

An abridged application may be made based on article 4.8a of directive 65/65/EEC ('on the approximation of provisions laid down by law, regulation or administrative action relating to proprietary medicinal products'). This allows a marketing authorization to be granted on the basis of essential similarity between the generic product and the originator.

Part I of an abridged marketing authorization application should provide the date of first authorization of the originator product and proof of continual authorization for 10 years within the European Union. The summary of product characteristics and the patient information leaflet should reflect the originator labelling. Part I also contains expert reports, though they are often shorter in length than those provided for a full marketing authorization application.

The requirements for part II of the marketing authorization application are the same as for a new chemical entity. The pharmaceutical form and the excipients may differ from the originator product. Sufficient work must be carried out to assure the regulatory authority that the active ingredient is comparable to the originator in terms of the route of synthesis, the specification and the impurities. The company must also carry out stability tests on the generic product.

Part III of the dossier is minimal unless:

- the application is for a different dose from that used for the originator product
- an excipient has never been used before in a pharmaceutical product
- the compound has a different impurity profile compared with the originator compound, in which case appropriate pre-clinical testing would be needed.

If the application is for a new combination generic product or if it concerns use in a different target population compared with the originator, appropriate research work must be carried out.

Part IV usually contains bioavailability data comparing the generic product against the originator. It may not be necessary to provide bioavailability data if the company can justify why such studies were not performed.

Data from clinical trials are not needed unless the proposed marketing authorization refers to differences in use of the product compared with the originator, e.g:

- different dose or dose interval
- modified release formulation
- different population
- different indication.

Veterinary products

In addition to the usual pre-clinical and clinical sections, dossiers for veterinary products have sections on residues for food-producing animals and ecotoxicity. In addition, there are strict guidelines for the production of these data which involve studies that can be very expensive to carry out, with significant analytical development being required in most cases. The clinical section of the human product dossier may be more extensive than that of a veterinary product but overall a full veterinary dossier for a new chemical entity will be 14+ volumes of data.

As is the case with a human pharmaceutical product, part I of the veterinary dossier is made up of administrative data, summary of product characteristics and the expert reports.

There are four different expert reports for a veterinary dossier, which cover:

- chemistry and pharmacy
- safety
- residue documentation
- pre-clinical and clinical findings.

Part II of the dossier covers chemistry and pharmacy, as is the case for the dossier for a human pharmaceutical product, and the sections are more or less identical to those required for human medicines. Part III of the dossier for a veterinary product is made up of safety and residue documentation. Part IV covers pre-clinical and clinical documentation.

All novel veterinary products for food-producing animals have to go through the centralized procedure for approval in Europe but at present products for use in small animals are excluded from this procedure. Biotechnology products must also go through the centralized procedure. Mutual recognition is also now available for the majority of veterinary products.

The veterinary regulatory authority of the UK is the Veterinary Medicines Directorate (VMD). It is recognized as one of the strictest EU authorities but it is also helpful when used as the reference member state for mutual recognition or as rapporteur for the centralized procedure.

Medical devices

There are over 150 000 different types of medical device marketed in Europe, from sticking plaster to cardiac pacemakers, and there are many differences between drug and device registration. While the medicines legislation framework has been in place for many years, over 80% of device legislation did not exist in 1990. Major pieces of legislation are the Safe Medicines Act in the USA and the Medical Device Legislation in Europe.

Devices in Europe are regulated by three separate directives:

- the active implantable medical device directive
- the medical device directive
- the in vitro diagnostic medical device directive.

Sometimes it is difficult to decide whether a product is a device or a medicinal product. In the past a product may have been registered as a medicinal product in one country and a device in another. Some products were previously registered as medicinal drug products but are now covered by device legislation. In this situation companies have an option as to which route to use for registration.

Medical devices are classed in a number of ways and the strictest controls are applied to those which present the greatest risk to health and safety. Class 1 devices are low risk, class 2A and 2B are medium risk and class 3 are high risk. In the UK the authority which controls devices is the Medical Devices Agency which reports to the Secretary of State for Health.

Information for patients, advertising and labelling

Pharmaceutical companies have a responsibility to make certain information available to patients. This includes information which must appear on a product's labelling and in the pack insert or patient information leaflet (PIL).

Companies often have dedicated staff responsible for writing patient information leaflets. PILs must be consistent with the summary of product characteristics and the marketing authorization and should not be promotional. They should include all contraindications, precautions, warnings and side-effects, but they do not have to include all of the indications. Various studies have been done to investigate what patients understand most easily. It is generally accepted that the language used in PILs should be clear and, whenever possible, non-technical. Sentences should be short. A question and answer approach seems to work well.

The information that must appear on the labelling of a product includes the product name, i.e. the brand name followed by the generic name. It should also include the pharmaceutical form of the product and the amount of the active ingredient. All excipients that are known to have a recognized pharmacological action or adverse effect must be included on the labelling. In the case of injectables, topical or eye preparations, a list of all the excipients must be shown. Any special warnings in line with the marketing authorization must be stated. The expiry date, storage and disposal instructions and the marketing authorization holder's name and address must also be shown.

There are certain cases in which products are exempt from full labelling because they are too small. These include small containers and strips and blister packs.

All advertising of pharmaceutical products is controlled by legislation and by various codes of practice. In Europe, prescription only medicines may be advertised only to health professionals and not to patients. In the USA, however, direct-to-consumer advertising is now permitted. OTC products may be advertised quite freely to patients in Europe and elsewhere.

The European directive on the advertising of medicinal products for human use (92/28/EEC) lays down statutory requirements which, in the UK, are implemented in the Medicines Act. These requirements are reflected in the European Code of Practice for the Promotion of Medicines (European Federation of Pharmaceutical Industries' Associations). In the UK the ABPI Code of Practice for the Pharmaceutical Industry applies to the promotion of medicines to health professionals. Promotion of OTC products in the UK is covered by the Code of Standards of Advertising Practice for Over-the-Counter Medicines. This code is administered by the Proprietary Association of Great Britain (PAGB). Further information on codes of practice is given in Chapter 16.

Further Reading and websites

Cartwright A C, Matthews B R 1991 Pharmaceutical Product Licensing: – requirements for Europe Ellis Horwood, New York

Dunlop D 1967 The assessment of the safety of drugs and the role of government in their control. Journal of Clinical Pharmacology and Journal of New Drugs 7 (4): 184–192

Eur-Lex (European Union Law) website: http://europa.eu.int/eur-lex/en/index.html

European Agency for the Evaluation of Medicinal Products (EMEA) website: http://www.emea.eu.int

UK Department of Health website: http://www.doh.gov.uk/

UK Medicines Control Agency website: http://www.open.gov.uk/mca/

US Food and Drug Administration website: http://www.fda.gov/

Chapter 14

Developments in records and document management

Sandy Chalmers

Introduction

This chapter explains the theory and practices of records management and of the closely related discipline of document management and how they may be best applied to the pharmaceutical industry. It views these subjects in the light of very rapid developments in information technology and offers insights into how pharmaceutical processes can be improved through the application of these techniques.

Records management and document management are important and rapidly changing disciplines within the pharmaceutical industry and the skills involved seem to be merging with a whole range of activities being carried out by information and information technology professionals.

This chapter will introduce the principles of these practices as applied to the pharmaceutical industry and will illustrate some of the overlaps and issues arising. In addition, some of the new skills required for these disciplines will be identified.

Specifically, the following topics will be addressed:

- how professionals can operate within the changing regulatory and legislative framework
- how information technology can improve current practices and, in some cases, revolutionize established operations
- how modern record centres have to adjust to a mixed media environment
- how skills and knowledge should be developed to enhance the value to the organization.

Records and their relationships

Records management has many definitions but my preferred one is:

Records management is the management and control of an organization's records applied to their creation, organization, use, preservation, retention and destruction. (Wiggins 1990a)

Records can take the form of paper, microfilm, electronic, image, photographs, biological specimens, wax blocks and so on. However, records should not be confused with information, which is considered to be 'usable data'. Thus a record can be considered as a container for information.

By comparison, document management is the terminology normally used for manipulations of electronic documents within a repository and this topic will be dealt with more fully in a later section.

The main concern of records management is the capture and management of records, once finalized, through the active and inactive phases of their lifespan; indeed records managers tend to be more interested in the medium than in the information it contains (Wiggins 1990b), but with technology developments this situation will be changing.

The lifespan of a record is of critical importance to the records manager as this determines where the record should be located, its accessibility and security and its value to the company in terms of its legal admissibility or compliance with regulations. Any changes in media format will have consequences for its management.

Figure 14.1 shows the relationships of active and inactive records and gives some approximate values for storage times.

Records managed using such a scheme have several advantages for the organization. For example,

- staff can find records that otherwise could not have been located and hence better decisions are made and possible protection afforded in litigation cases
- staff can find records more quickly
- records are kept for an appropriate length of time rather than indefinitely, which saves either computer or physical space
- records organized properly will almost certainly make it easier to apply new technologies as needed.

Records will of course vary in their rate of production and complexity and can be as diverse as memos and emails to compilations such as regulatory submissions. Examples will be given in the sections below.

Regulatory environment

Within the pharmaceutical industry, there are many regulatory, legal and statutory obligations that are imposed on records and their handling and these will be described below. In addition, companies may wish to work to their own standards in areas which are unaffected by these obligations, to ensure the validity of their research or the admissibility of records involving the organization's intellectual property. Thus the records manager may have to apply a wide range of controls on records depending on their origin and use. For instance, in the early stages of research where an active substance is being identified, management of laboratory data, e.g. analytical data, spectra, experimental notes etc., will be essential from the intellectual property point of view.

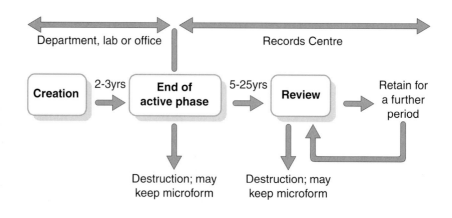

Figure 14.1
Relationships of active and inactive records

The subsequent phases of product development are governed by specific regulations which must be accommodated to allow a drug entity to progress to manufacture and sale. These are as follows:

- pre-clinical toxicity testing—Good Laboratory Practice (GLP)
- clinical trials—Good Clinical Practice (GCP)
- manufacture—Good Manufacturing Practice (GMP).

Each of the phases has its own controls on the records and the way they are produced. Regulatory authority monitoring units can inspect an organization's operations and facilities including records management and archiving procedures. The implications of this are described below.

Good Laboratory Practice

GLP aims to ensure that, as far as possible, the quality and integrity of laboratory non-clinical raw data (Statutory Instrument 1997) meet the required standards. The derived records must be managed in the laboratories and record centres to agreed high standards of safety and security; internal auditing of studies helps to ensure quality of these processes.

The raw data exists in a wide variety of media, e.g. from paper through to magnetic media etc. Once experimentation is completed by the user department and the data reported, the records need to be directed to a secure area with controlled access. This physically secure area will have access to it controlled by trained records management staff and the processes for storing, retrieving, viewing and copying records will be documented in Standard Operating Procedures (SOPs).

Typical records would include study files, toxicology reports, formulation records, laboratory notes, traces, certificates, biological specimens, wax blocks, histology slides, reserve samples, chromatograms, stability records etc.

If records have to be amended or updated, a clear process for doing this must exist. Any changes must be signed and explained. Thus all changes of any kind need to be documented in full.

These records are inspectable by the relevant regulatory authorities, e.g. the Food and Drug Administration (FDA) or the Medicines Control Agency (MCA). Inspections take place on a regular basis; however specific inspections may occur at any time for a particular study or product. During any inspections, records are expected to be delivered to the inspectors with minimum delay and SOPs, training records, job descriptions, organization charts etc. are usually high on the inspector's list for viewing in addition to selected studies. The inspectors are looking not only for complete, authentic records of the work done and the procedures involved but evidence that users are working to these documented procedures.

The use of electronic signatures in the GLP context is an important development and the FDA has issued a Final Rule on the subject. This will be dealt with in a later section on Emergent Technology.

Good Clinical Practice

GCP ensures that clinical trial data is managed to high scientific and ethical standards and includes the requirement to maintain records to demonstrate this. The responsibilities of the sponsor (company), trial monitors and trial investigators are defined in the GCP rules, among these being the obligation to ensure accuracy, safety and the archiving of relevant trial records. An overview (Rammell 1997) offers insights into the practicalities of operating to GCP standards and cross-refers to efforts to harmonize clinical trial processes in the European Union, United States and Japan in the form of ICH principles (ICH 1996).

A large number of record types (over 50) are created during the clinical trial process, these records being created before, during and after the clinical phase. Some examples of these are investigators' brochures, protocols and amendments, certificates of analysis, case report forms, informed consent forms, monitors' visit reports, audit certificates and many more. These records have to be carefully handled and stored as part of GCP duties. The regulations clarify which record types the investigator and sponsor should hold and many of the standards identified earlier in GLP apply to GCP as well.

Good Manufacturing Practice

The UK Medicines Act requires that a licence is acquired prior to manufacture of a pharmaceutical product. To obtain this licence, an organization has to demonstrate that the manufacturing processes and the attendant records are up to a standard as required by GMP regulations (Medicines Control Agency 1997). These define standards for quality, safety and efficacy of the product and are based on the facilities in use (premises, plant, equipment), staff (qualifications, authority) and procedural records.

Many of the record types encountered in GMP relate to analytical and quality control and include material specifications, manufacturing formula and processing instructions, batch processing records, batch packaging records, procedures, laboratory notebooks, environmental data, validation records, calibration records etc.

The basic requirements for records handling are documented elsewhere (Kendall 1996) but as with the other good practices described above, a rigorous trail of records is needed to substantiate what was done, why it was done and by whom, and any deviations from standard practice. Regulatory authorities can and do make inspections and, because manufacturing may be ongoing at the time of the inspection, inspectors may view GMP manufacturing practices during the visit.

Legal issues

As with any industry, there are a number of legal and statutory records which a pharmaceutical company must hold to be able to function in a business environment. These aspects will not be addressed here (Emmerson 1989); however, litigation cases in the pharmaceutical industry are increasingly common and a company can find itself bound by law to produce evidence in support or in defence of a court case.

Three types of litigation cases are common:

- patent litigation: alleged invalidity or infringement of intellectual property rights
- product litigation: alleged harmful effects of drugs/devices etc.
- safety litigation: alleged workplace health issues.

In some of these cases, the company may have to supply many thousands of records to a court as part of a so-called document discovery process. The company is obliged to find all records on a certain topic or product and this task is much assisted if a records system is in place where the records can be readily searched for and located. Records on all types of media are required and this will include letters, memos, minutes of meetings, batch records, reports etc. and also email, faxes, optical images, samples etc. The task is quite daunting for the records manager who may be coordinating the project within various departments.

Interestingly, in litigations, location and supply of superseded (but at one time valid) records can be important. This is because what was in operation at the time of the event causing the litigation may be considered important rather than what is currently known (retention strategies will be dealt with below).

Needless to say, litigation cases are usually very costly and can run into millions of pounds or dollars. It should be stressed that an effective records management system, which can identify milestone events and can help to piece together the chronology of decisions on product history, can be very valuable to the organization.

In this context, aspiring records or document managers should be aware of the clear distinction between information and evidence in such cases. Information may or may not identify when it was originated, by whom and in what context. Evidence on the other hand, usually contains a date and often a signature or some equivalent verification of the author. With certain criteria being met, the record may be admissible as evidence in court; however, there may still be some doubt about the actual credibility and authenticity of the record and hence the weight of evidence needs to be assessed in court for the record to be believed (Smith 1996). Indeed the credibility of the witness may be called into question; for example is the witness qualified, trained and competent to use computer systems? Thus although many of the modern information technologies offer a wide range of information to the user, the use of some of these technologies as evidence in the court room still has to be assessed. A useful initiative in such matters is the British Standard Institution Code of Practice (1999), which identifies good practices for managing information on electronic storage media, e.g. WORM and CD-ROM as well as rewritable media, and greatly helps to support records as legally admissible and of high evidential value.

A balance is clearly required where critical records need to be available as evidence (in whatever form), with other records readily accessible as information for business operations.

Practices

Audits and surveys

In order to assess how any particular department organizes and handles its records, a records manager must propose some kind of investigation of the processes involved. If he/she wishes to check against an agreed and established procedure, an audit should be conducted. If he/she were trying to assess what staff are currently doing, then a survey would give an understanding of the types and volumes of records in use; it would also provide indication of the nomenclature for records which the department uses, how the records are stored and how long they are kept, their security and confidentiality and their copying and onward transmissions. Being able to collect this information greatly assists in compliance with retention schedules, with regulatory requirements and in redesign projects or any other similar initiatives.

Carrying out such an audit or survey requires considerable planning and resources. A project proposal should be developed by first gaining the commitment of a high level sponsor and the full cooperation of the user department where resources may be needed. Good ongoing communications with the department during the project are essential as well as regular review of progress, this helping to keep the project in focus.

Conducting the survey may be done in several ways depending on the type of department and the spectrum of records involved. Some techniques are shown in Table 14.1.

Once the data has been collected and analysed, it is often useful to get verification of the data from a user representative to ensure no misunderstandings have arisen. Reporting back to the department with conclusions and recommendations often needs to be handled with considerable care but is very important as the delivery style and impact could markedly affect the effectiveness of the implementation of new practices.

Retention scheduling

Retaining records for a specified length of time before either destroying them or at least reviewing them for possible destruction is not a new concept. However, setting the period of

*Table 14.1   Survey
techniques*

Advantages	Disadvantages
Questionnaires:	
Standard questions and answers lead to ready evaluation	Response rate may be variable
Large groups accommodated	No flexibility in each answer
Easy distribution (hard copy or electronic)	
Face-to-face interviews:	
Questions can be discussed and clarified	Time consuming
All questions will be answered	Easy to digress into other issues
May get some extra information	
Focus groups:	
Save time	Require careful selection of members
Consensus feedback	May be difficult to arrange
Physical survey:	
View of real situation	Time consuming
Physical limitations and technology observed	Staff may feel threatened

retention for certain records is sometimes difficult to do and is dependent on a number of issues.

In some cases, for instance financial records, there is a statutory requirement to retain records for a certain time and there is little debate needed. In other cases, a regulatory authority may require a minimum retention time and this will be discussed in more detail below. However, in other cases, an organization can choose which length of time it deems correct and this is usually based on litigation or scientific research needs. This is often perceived as a kind of insurance and is determined by assessing risks in a fairly crude sort of way. Often the question arises: when does it become more costly to retain the record in terms of storage and access than its possible value?

Another issue centres on the point on which a retention time should start. In simple cases, the date of issue of the record is the trigger but with records which are compiled over time, e.g. bound laboratory notebooks, project files etc., there may be a period of six months or more from the starting of the record to its completion. In these cases it is safer to work from the completion date so that all parts of the record meet a minimum retention time.

In regulated areas, the situation may be even more complicated and may depend on whether the drug reaches the dossier submission and marketplace stages. If the drug does not reach the market, the end of study date is usually the important one and regulatory authority minimum times, as per the territory, apply. Where the drug does reach the market, the trigger is based on the date of approval of the marketing application in the particular region, but additional constraints are described in ICH GCP Guidelines 1996.

Another factor in this discussion is around compliance with the agreed retention times. Do companies have the time and inclination to spend effort in identifying records at expiry of the retention period, seeking the owner's review and possible approval for destruction and then arranging destruction? What is the situation when an originator of a set of records leaves the company or retires—who takes ownership? All these questions require quite stringent procedures to be in place for the process to work effectively.

Some organizations find it easier to work to a 'destruction' retention period, i.e. once the time period is completed the record is automatically destroyed without any final review and approval. This means that the retention period has to be clearly identified at the birth of the record but in some cases it may be difficult to assess whether the record will have value at the end of its assigned period.

Another issue arises around when the records centre should actually receive records. In GLP areas, the policy preferred by authorities is to have the records secured in a safe, controlled place as soon as the records are complete and, where necessary, signed off. In contrast, in non-regulated areas, staff usually prefer to let the record become inactive or semi-inactive before the record is 'archived'. This may also relate to the fact that certain records are batched together with other similar records prior to the 'archiving process' and hence delays occur. Nevertheless, the retention time should operate from the date of origin of the record not the time at which it was sent to the records centre.

The records manager will also meet issues particular to electronic records. Unlike hard copy records that occupy physical space and can be seen to be building up, electronic records are much more 'invisible' and tend to be forgotten even if they do have a retention period associated with them. The database then gets cluttered up with out-of-date records and its efficiency diminishes. Some kind of electronic alert to the expiry of the retention time needs to be embedded into the system.

The detail of retention scheduling strategies can be read elsewhere (Emmerson 1989). One of the traps that records managers fall into is managing the records by their names and formats rather than by their true series. For instance, are laboratory notebooks managed in the same way as electronic or loose-leaf laboratory notes? Records should not be managed by convenience but by their true business value and records managers must face this challenge.

One other point to be made is that, despite diverse views from departments, the organization should reach corporate agreement on retention times and documented standards for each series produced. Such documentation gives the opportunity to record any justified deviations from standard policy and allows users to understand the process and their obligations more fully.

Storage

Physical storage

Historically, most effort has been put into storing and preserving hard copy records and microfilm; suitable standards have been established to protect these materials over long periods of time (see Stockford 1996 for microfilm standards). In records management terms, although the records are not normally retained for extended periods, the standards of temperature control and humidity etc. are still of good value; a range of other protections (Kitching 1993) should also be recognized, e.g. pest control measures, gas suppression systems to extinguish fires, water detectors to alert staff to flooding etc.

In terms of security, an organization should invest in a separate, secure storage area (a records centre) with trained resident staff to control access and to manage activities such as record receipt, indexing, storage, retrieval, copying, consultation and distribution. The design of the buildings and the means of storage, e.g. mobile shelving units, can be found in Kitching 1993. Where space allows, a separate reading area is a desirable facility where records can be delivered to the user for consultation; users should not have unaccompanied access to any area other than the reading area and, in the case of a regulated records centre, their visits would be recorded.

In considering storage, an organization needs to determine whether an on-site or off-site storage facility (or both) is required. This cannot be treated in depth here but use of an external contract company providing storage and retrieval services may be of value to the business. Clearly, the level of service required, e.g. the frequency of deliveries to and from the contract facility, the speed of access, the level of indexing and computerization and the likelihood of regulatory inspections are all factors that need to be taken into consideration.

Coupled with these decisions are the issues of disaster planning. Is there a risk that whole collections either in record centres or in departments may suffer total loss to fire, flooding or explosion? Duplicating large collections is not normally practical but making an assessment of the organization's information assets and duplicating the vital sets on a separate site may be a good strategy. Indeed, separating duplicate sets may be an alternative to high levels of protection of a single set and may be more cost effective than installing gas protection systems etc. However, as more and more collections are available electronically, electronic duplication is likely to be the best protection.

Electronic storage

The technology of storage of electronic and image records is a highly specialized subject and will not be dealt with here. However, the use of such facilities to store and manage records is clearly a developing activity and strategies are discussed below.

The term 'electronic archiving' is now in common use but, for those involved in managing records, it should not be confused with computer backup techniques; the latter is a very important operation to ensure that data and information are not lost in the event of an emergency. Electronic archiving on the other hand is a predetermined operation to store inactive electronic records in a format and location from which they can easily be retrieved.

Of major importance to the records manager is the logical access to stored electronic records—who should be able to store records, have access, change records, copy records etc? The fact that electronic records are easily changed poses problems over the authenticity of the record as well as creating confusion over the possibility of a variety of different versions being available. The records manager has a part to play in introducing the disciplines of good practices here.

One approach (Chalmers & Purdue 1996) was to develop a regulated electronic archiving system in parallel with the GLP paper system in which electronic files were manipulated like paper ones and transferred either :

- to the control of records centre staff who ensure the change control, retention, location requirements as needed for GLP compliance, or
- automatically via a security interface which could control access rights, thus complying with GLP requirements (Fig. 14.2).

This is perhaps the first step towards establishing more sophisticated repositories where users can be responsible for transferring their own records into an electronic storage area which could be secured to GLP standards of change control.

As noted above, there are now many different kinds of media that comprise records. Each may have its own advantage to the organization. For example, paper and microform are relatively cheap and difficult to falsify but have the disadvantage of being cumbersome to revise where this is necessary. With the rapid development of software upgrades, electronic media may suffer from technology redundancy and the records manager has to decide whether to continually upgrade to current software systems or to convert to more 'stable'

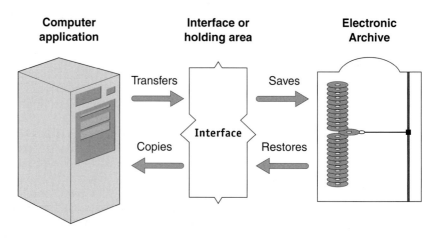

Figure 14.2 *Electronic archiving system*

media. Some media will comprise legacy systems where the cost of converting to different media is prohibitive; others will be concerned with legal admissibility of one form being preferred over another. Thus for the records manager the issue is how to manage all of these media simultaneously and this is clearly a challenge.

Protection of confidentiality

The physical protection of records has been referred to above. However, a further question arises: does every record need the same confidentiality protection? The answer is clearly no, but the strategy for achieving this grading of protection is harder to implement. Linked to this is the concept of confidentiality where the protection is not against loss, fire and flood but from disclosure to parties who have no need nor rights to see the records.

One solution is to classify records into different categories and to implement protections on each level according to its value. The following is a general description of one approach:

- highly confidential—very sensitive material
- company confidential—intellectual assets
- standard—general office records
- for public viewing—journal, patent articles.

Following such a scheme preserves advantage over competitors, avoids over-protection of many records, saves costs and gives a consistent graded protection across the organization.

Associated with these four levels are a number of information classification controls which would need to be implemented, e.g. markings on the record to indicate which class it belongs to, who can have access, who can have copies, different means of disposal of records, security on mailings, controls on email and faxes etc.

Clearly, to make this work, staff would have to develop a discipline for the management of the records at these different levels. Staff education and training as well as feedback sessions and even audits will be essential.

Related to confidentiality, the protection of personally identifiable data in the pharmaceutical environment is becoming a considerable issue. The electronic manipulation now possible with modern computer techniques opens up databases containing personal data to possible intentional or unintentional abuse. ICH GCP rules are clear on the importance of confidentiality and privacy during clinical trials and the advent of new European legislation (European Directive 1995), effective from October 1998 has brought the views on human rights to the fore. European states are in the process of converting this framework directive into their own national legislations, this allowing for a basic set of harmonized principles to apply throughout the European Economic Area. The impact of this legislation for non-EEA countries is currently being assessed.

The principles of the new legislation are described briefly below. Personal data should be:

- processed fairly and lawfully
- for explicit purposes and not further processed in a way incompatible with those purposes
- adequate and not excessive
- accurate and up to date
- kept for a minimum time.

A number of issues for the pharmaceutical industry have arisen, the three main ones being as follows:

Consent

Consent for processing of a data subject's personal information is a critical feature and, for prospective studies, obtaining consent should be incorporated in the pre-study procedures.

However there are a number of healthcare related areas where consent is either difficult or impossible to obtain, e.g. pharmaco-epidemiology, cancer registers etc. The pharmaceutical industry is in debate with authorities to agree exemptions in these areas.

The data subject's right of access and right to object

The new legislation has given much more extensive rights to the individual as far as accessing data and having inaccuracies rectified, defining consent etc. Much needs to be done to ensure that there is a balance between the patient's rights and the free flowing of medical research.

Transfer of personal data to and from Europe

Perhaps the most controversial aspect of the new legislation is the restriction of personal data being transferred to a country which does not have 'adequate' data protection. The topic is too complex for discussion here but resolution of the problems particularly between the EU and the US needs to be achieved to avoid international trade issues.

Resolving these and other issues is clearly of a high priority and the trade organizations in Europe (EFPIA, European Federation of Pharmaceutical Industries and Associations) and US (PhRMA, Pharmaceutical Research and Manufacturers of America) are actively trying to facilitate agreement.

Policies

Whatever control over records is needed, a company needs to demonstrate how it handles its records in a documented way. This may be in the form of a policy, procedure or manual etc., but it is beneficial for an organization to have a clear understanding of the roles of these different documentations which govern the management of the records. Distinction between these and their impact on records management has been detailed (Chalmers 1998) but the following definitions give a basic clarification:

- Policy: A high level statement of fundamentals that need to be achieved, i.e. a statement of intent or position describing agreed course or action.
- Procedure: A document describing a process critical to achieving high product quality or regulatory or statutory compliance.
- Standard: A clearly defined minimum level of quality that must be achieved and against which all procedures and guidelines should comply.
- Guideline: A description of recommended best practice for a process or activity but which may not be mandatory.

Demarcation of documents as in Figure 14.3 will help organizations to clarify practices for their users, particularly identifying when they are mandatory and when optional. This leads to more consistent practices across the company and helps to improve efficiency.

Emergent technology

The rapid growth and sophistication of computer technology have a large impact on many records management operations. A records manager has to think in new ways and be able to accommodate both the basic requirements of hardcopy collections and evolving dynamic records coming from software systems.

Electronic mail (email) for instance has revolutionized the work patterns of most of us and an account of the typical features of a system can be read elsewhere (Bronson 1998). Not only do the emails themselves proliferate, but electronic documents attached to the email

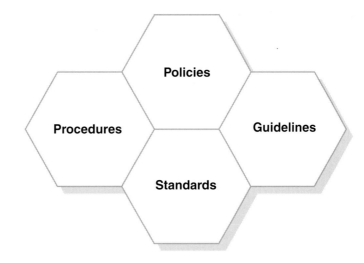

Figure 14.3
Document demarcation

add to the complexity by 'hiding' within the text. What was originally conceived as a means of communications is often being used as a storage system, for which it is ill-suited and is not cost-effective.

In addition, with the ease of use of email, many users have become poorly disciplined and do not actively manage their email records to any great extent. Folders fill up, locating specific emails becomes harder and there are often no retention times associated with them. Not only do business processes suffer but the risk in litigation cases becomes quite substantial since many emails may be written without background or qualification and may be quoted out of context in court cases.

The records manager therefore should have a role in the education and training of users to ensure they control their emails in a manageable way. As an aid to this, an email janitor could be invaluable; this would automatically delete records after an agreed time period, based on the date of last modification of the record. Normally, a short period such as a week is given before absolute destruction, in case the user has a last minute need to retain a significant record. In-file, out-file and unread emails would each have standard agreed retention times.

Another aspect of email education is to change the culture of the users in order to manage their email better and thus save on computing resources. For instance, users should :

- not distribute emails widely unless absolutely necessary
- use attachments sparingly (use shared areas instead, where possible)
- not reply to all recipients if not appropriate.

Equal to the pre-eminence of email is the use of the internet/intranet and its features are described elsewhere (Mathers 1997). It has become an excellent awareness tool and has in addition the attraction of use of graphics and animation. It relies however on the user going to look for the information rather than the traditional route of information being sent to the desk of the user. This should not be a real problem but demands a change in user culture.

Where the internet/intranet is less impressive is in the following aspects:

- quoted URLs seem to go out of date quite quickly and may not always be useful to cross-reference records
- the security of the firewalls is normally good but is not infallible
- the legal admissibility of records held on an organization's intranet is under debate; authenticity and change control are areas of weakness.

Thus the advantage of dynamic records for speed of issue and awareness has a downside in terms of authenticity and reliability. The role for the records manager is to assess how the best of these aspects can be accommodated.

In other technology areas, the records manager can be helped by using records management software, i.e. software which is specifically designed to support records management processes such as:

- registering the existence of records
- recording information about records
- prompting the user to do things with records
- tracking what has been done to records
- producing documentation which controls records, e.g. lists, reports, labels
- providing management information on a range of activities.

Software systems may well address several of these functions but are unlikely to cover all of them. Systems can be used to record and track the transactions between physical locations and electronic sites so that the status of the record and its related information can be made available at any time. Typical routings would be from the user's PC to a records centre, a user's filing system or an off-site storage site/destruction site.

As with many software applications, the technologies are changing rapidly and information on each technology needs to be kept up to date (Parker 1998). However, of equal importance are the modifications in the customer demands for records management (and hence changes to the systems) and it is an ongoing task for the records manager to keep aware of changes in the business needs. Also changes in regulations and standards may be thrust upon the records manager and alterations to the software will need to be made to accommodate these.

Once the functionality of a records management system has been identified, the next task is to decide how to develop it. Perhaps an in-house development may be possible, or making use of an already established application by modifying it. Another alternative is to buy an off-the-shelf specialist package.

There are no guidelines to determine which of these options is best, this being dependent on the merits of each case. However, validation of the system to ensure that it performs correctly and to the standard required is essential.

No discussion of electronic records would be complete without some reference to the developing use of electronic signatures within the industry. Consideration of the use of electronic signatures in electronic records originated in the early 1990s from US discussions on how to improve the efficiency of manufacturing practices. The aim was to streamline operations and to speed up reviews and approvals, while at the same time stopping fraudulent practices. After much consultation, the FDA issued a Final Rule in the March 1997 Federal Register which allowed electronic alternatives to hand-written signatures for manufacturing and regulatory purposes under certain controlled conditions. The signatures can be biometric (eg. fingerprints, eye retinae etc) or non-biometric (identification code plus password) and must conform to certain rules including ensuring that the signatures are bound to the respective records to avoid any possible 'cutting and pasting' of signatures. Details can be found in the Final Rule or in the paper by Dietz et al 1998.

Although the Final Rule became effective in August 1997, its application has been mainly limited to manufacturing areas and wider use within GLP and GCP areas has been slow to date. However, as expertise develops, electronic signatures will no doubt have an important place in future electronic record management systems.

Document management

So far most of this chapter has been concerned with records management. This section will now address the concept of document management that in its broadest sense can cover any management of a document, e.g. a database of images or electronic text etc. However, the definition more commonly used particularly by IT specialists is as follows:

Document management is the efficient and effective production, storage, retrieval and dissemination of documents and information from which they are compiled to achieve maximum business benefits.

Document management nowadays nearly always means electronic document management and commonly refers to managing 'active' documents; the term 'document' itself is quite difficult to define but can often be described in the traditional way of having a recognizable start and end, and usually text in the middle; in contrast, a record does not need to have these attributes!

It is to be noted that a wide variety of optical-based storage systems are called document management systems; these vary in features but most often are images of documents scanned onto optical storage devices which offer quick and convenient access to the whole text of a document and are much more versatile than the equivalent paper collection held at a single location.

However, the focus here will concern the workflow aspects of the electronic document lifespan, i.e. the creation, drafting, review, approval, distribution, storage, revision and change control of each stage. Figure 14.4 shows this graphically.

Manipulating electronic versions of documents in a controlled way has a number of benefits :

- a single electronic version can be shared within the business around different sites
- ability to undertake full-text retrieval of the document
- staff can more easily re-use parts of documents and modify them if necessary
- documents can be communicated externally to the organization
- regulatory rules can be met more easily
- a higher quality of final output is achieved.

Re-use of information within a document, such as a submission compilation, is a very important factor for saving time and reducing tedious paperwork tasks. Thus the produc-

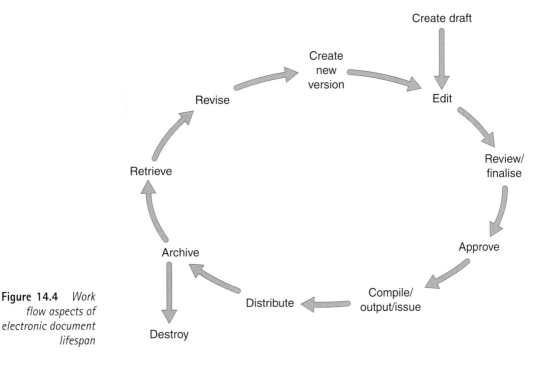

Figure 14.4 *Work flow aspects of electronic document lifespan*

Create draft

Create new version

Edit

Revise

Review/finalise

Retrieve

Approve

Archive

Compile/output/issue

Distribute

Destroy

tion of the following typical submission documents can be directly affected by improvements in document management:

- CTX : Clinical Trials Exemption
- IND : Investigational New Drug Application
- NDA : New Drug Application
- MAA : Marketing Authorization Application

For several years, the production of these submissions has been under pressure from factors such as too much paper being produced and too little space to store the component documents as well as the resultant submission. Added to this, incompatible formats, misplaced information and last minute alterations have slowed the production rate and raised the possibility of introducing errors. Hence, document management, integrated with other technological advances such as groupware, workflow and image processing has had a significant effect on the efficiency and effectiveness of the submission process. Figure 14.5 shows a generic document management architecture.

In order to ensure that the component parts of a submission are able to be brought together like pieces of a jigsaw, a set of standards needs to be agreed for the formats of the components. This will include defining text and table font sizes, page layout features such as margins, heading styles, indentations, text justifications and pagination. In addition, the management of tables within the text and nomenclature for trade marks, compound names and numbers etc. need to be agreed and adhered to by the users. Clearly in this area, the promotion of policies and standards for staff is essential.

A focus for the page layout and format is of course the use of standard templates; these can be of huge benefit by building into the template a number of features which will help

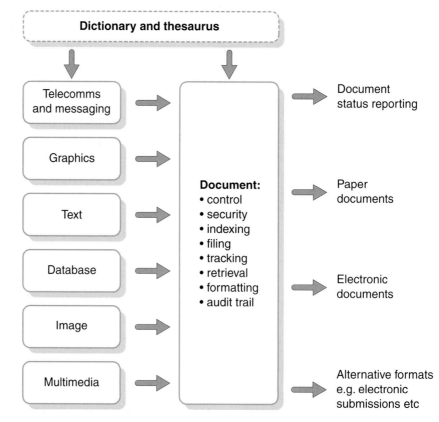

Figure 14.5 *Generic document management architecture*

the author to concentrate on the intellectual aspects of the content rather than the detail of the format. For instance, the template can include so-called 'boilerplate text' which is standard text appearing in every document of that type; the author then needs to add the specific text for that particular document. Also available can be colour-coded help text which indicates to the author when to insert certain sections or paragraphs or when to replace already formatted dummy fields with real text. Separate electronic guidance may be required to give the author high-level assistance in the use of these templates.

Use of such templates greatly enhances the look and feel of the resultant compilation and encourages sharing and re-use of sections of information. Ultimately the navigation of the documentation is improved, which may in turn lead to speedier approvals.

Other features which can be built into these templates are metadata values. These vary from values such as document numbers, dates and authors to confidentiality classification fields, signature fields, copyright etc. Some of these, if standardized, greatly assist in information retrieval and version control of the documents. The latter is extremely important in document management as multiple versions of very similar documents are a major source of errors. Version identifiers for each version can be built into the document number but the author is faced with the question as to what constitutes a change to a document and will it require the creation of a completely new version; the reason can vary from a typographical error to a revision of an entire section. Rationalization of these issues and implementation of policies are some of the challenges for the records manager.

Redesign

The speeding up of the submission process is the goal of many research-based pharmaceutical companies. Redesigning the process so that the submission is broken down into smaller sub-document units which can be recombined to form a variety of outputs is an approach being developed by Glaxo Wellcome. These units, called modules, are first identified from an information plan derived from research, development and commercial interests and are constructed using customized templates and guides. They can range in granularity from a paragraph to a whole document and are stored in electronic form in a version-controlled repository where they are available for use. Authorized staff can access the information in these 'building block' modules at a much earlier stage than previously and can use them to build other enlarged modules. When the required modules are complete, they are approved for release and combined to give various outputs which are transformed using publishing software into submission material.

The benefits of such an approach are significant; the process encourages staff to make module information available at a much earlier time and to re-use and redistribute information efficiently. The culture of individuals hoarding information in their own areas is being changed to a more sharing environment where completed documents are readily available and are built more quickly.

A significant thought for the records manager is the question: in the future will many more document types be created in this way, i.e. built up according to a plan from component parts? If so, each component will have an existence similar to a document; will this mean that the records or document manager will have to control the lifespan of the modules in the same way as is done with documents and records? I believe it will.

Electronic submissions

The development of electronic submissions has been ongoing for some years and is considered a very desirable goal as it would mean:

■ shorter approval times as the submission would be more easily navigated and data more readily analysed
■ enhanced ability to retrieve information compared with previously submitted dossiers

- Has the scope been identified? Which sites and departments are participating?
- Is the team too small? (not enough representation)
- Is the team too large? (too many different views!)
- Are the team members empowered? (do they have the power to act for the department?)
- Does the team approve or recommend? And will senior management accept the decisions made?

Once these questions have been satisfied and, assuming senior management has been kept aware of progress and relevant feedback, and is assured that subordinate staff are committed to the initiative, the RD Manager may seek final senior management approval.

Implementation of the project will be the next phase and the immediate question will be whether a pilot is to be run or whether the new system will operate in parallel with the old one. The resources involved, including maintenance, need to be identified.

Once an initiative has been implemented, the RD Manager may need to supply metrics on the new benefits of the practices. These quality measures may sometimes be difficult to define or quantify but are nevertheless very important to demonstrate value to the business.

The personal qualities which would assist the RD Manager are harder to specify and may depend on the organizational structure and culture. However an ability to organize will be important as well as an outward-going personality. Being meticulous is often quoted as a prime requirement but only if the person remains objective at the same time. Hopefully this will ensure that the person will not get lost in detail and will be able to fulfil the task.

Adopting a proactive approach within the RD Manager role is critical. Trends and issues must be recognized at as early a stage as possible and acted upon. This proactivity can take the form of raising awareness with staff or departments or of preliminary investigations, but where there is an issue, the situation must not be allowed to develop without some action on the part of the RD Manager.

Conclusion

Considering all the topics in this chapter, one must surely come to the conclusion that there are many challenges for the aspiring RD Manager. For someone equipped with the above skills, the following will offer considerable personal development:

- management of electronic records to meet legal and regulatory needs
- development of electronic document systems to replace paper systems
- understanding and influencing users in how they manage records
- analysis of practices and definitions of procedures and policies to ensure compliance
- managing the multimedia scene
- making retention schedules work!

References

British Standards Institution 1999 Code of practice for legal admissibility and evidential weight of information stored electronically. DISC PD0008

Bronson K 1998 Managing e-mail in today's company. Records Management Bulletin 87 (August): 29–33

Chalmers A M 1998 Managing corporate records and standards on a global basis. Records Management Bulletin 87 (August): 66–67

Chalmers A M, Purdue C J R 1996 Electronic data archiving in a regulated environment. The International Records Management Journal 9(1): 14–18

Code of Federal Register 1997 Electronic records, electronic signatures. 21 CFR Part11

Dietz C, Nelson J, Salazar J 1998 New FDA regulations using computer technology. Pharmaceutical Engineering 18(1): 32–38

Emmerson P 1989 How to manage your records. ICSA Publishing, Cambridge

European Parliament and Council 1995 Directive 95/46/EC of the European Parliament and of the Council: On the protection of individuals with regard to the processing of personal data and on the free movement of such data. EC, Luxembourg. http://europa.eu.int/eur-lex/en/lif/dat/1995/en_395L0046.html

International Conference on Harmonization 1996 ICH harmonized tripartite guideline for good clinical practice. ICH Secretariat, Geneva

Kendall V 1996 Good manufacturing practices for pharmaceutical products. Scrip Report, PJB Publications, Richmond

Kitching C 1993 HMSO archive buildings in UK 1977–1992. HMSO, London

Marr A P 1998 Electronic submissions—what's the future. The Regulatory Review 3 (April): 3–7

Mathers J 1997 Using the internet. Records Management Bulletin 79: 9–14

Medicines Control Agency 1997 Rules and guidance for pharmaceutical manufacturers and distributors. The Stationary Office, London

Parker E 1998 Records management software survey. Records Management Bulletin 4 (February)

Rammell E 1997 The trials of clinical records management: Making sense of GCP. Records Management Bulletin 81 (August): 3–5

Smith G J H 1996 Imaging—Admissibility and other legal issues. BSI Conference of Legal Admissibility and Code of Practice, Manchester, March

Statutory Instrument 1997 Health and safety. Good laboratory practice regulations; 1997: no. 654. The Stationery Office, London

Stockford B 1996 Microfilm—a useful tool. Records Management Bulletin 76 (October): 23–30

Wiggins R E 1990a Information management. Records Management Bulletin 40 (October): 3–7

Wiggins R E 1990b Information management. Records Management Bulletin 39 (August): 3–7

Further Reading

British Standards Institution 1995 British standard code of practice for information security management. (BS 7799) and Guide (DISC PD0007).

Pease J 1995 Setting up a GCP archive. Records Management Bulletin 66 (February): 9–10

Penn I A, Pennix G, Coulson J 1994 Records management handbook, 2nd edn. Gower Publishing, Aldershot

Stephens D O 1998 Megatrends in records management. Records Management Bulletin 86 (June): 3–9

Chapter 15

End-user support and training

Elisabeth Goodman with contribution from Geraldine Boyce

Introduction

The range and sophistication of desktop information resources available today present scientists, clinicians, other health professionals, technical and business staff with a wide choice of options for meeting their information requirements. Yet today, as in the 1970s and '80s, we still raise the question of how much end-users should be encouraged to do their own searching, as opposed to using the skills of information professionals.

This chapter describes the issues associated with end-user searching. It refers mainly to the pharmaceutical industry but the concepts apply to other organizations and services. In it we discuss the user-friendly features of a 'state-of-the-art' desktop resource; the emerging role of information professionals in relation to end-users; and approaches for training and supporting end-users.

Who is the end-user of information?

Definitions and history—the context for the present day

In a 1996 article entitled 'End-users: they come and grow', the author (Ghilhardi 1996) makes two points which reoccur consistently in discussions on end-user searching:

- it takes time for end-users to search, especially if they are unfamiliar with the sources
- for Ghilhard's company, end-user searching resulted in more (not less) work for the information professionals.

'End-users' are commonly referred to as individuals without formal qualification or expertise in the searching of electronic bibliographic databases (usually external). Much of the published literature on this subject refers to this context.

Our own experience in the pharmaceutical industry extends beyond external, bibliographic databases, to all electronic sources of information, be they internal or external, bibliographic references, full text articles, data or reports. When we come on to discuss the changing role of information specialists, training and support, it is this wider context that we will be addressing.

What are their needs?

When to be an end-user versus using an intermediary

As long ago as 1970, Bennett (1970) raised questions relating to the viability of direct end-user/machine interaction which, in one form or another, are still being raised today:

- Can a system be designed for use by the general public?
- What are the characteristics of the users served by the facility?
- What are the problems in the education and training of the end-user?
- What are the operational characteristics of the facilities that place constraints on use by the end-users?
- Is the assumption that end-users are less motivated to do their own searching a valid one?
- Will the end-user use the facility often enough to gain expertise in the use of the system?
- Will the end-user use the system enough to make it cost-effective?

Since 1970 there has been an enormous amount of literature on these themes, and some useful reviews (Eisenberg 1983, Nicholas & Harman 1985, Ting-Ming 1988, Walker 1988).

Charles Meadow wrote a pivotal paper on end-user searching in 1979, in which he stated that intermediaries had 'the keys to the kingdom' and often behaved accordingly (Meadow 1979). He predicted that intermediaries would spend less time 'hand-holding' and more time 'problem-solving'.

This section addresses each of Bennett's questions in turn. (For 'general public' read 'end-user'.)

Can a system be designed for use by the general public?

Although end-user systems can and have been designed, only some people (between 30% and 65%) will choose to use them on a more or less regular basis. Figures tend to drop off after the initial surge resulting from publicity and training (Cornick 1989, Dedert & Johnson 1990, Mischo & Lee 1987, Sewell & Teitelbaum 1986, Summitt 1989, Whittall 1988). Conversely, end-user searching of CAS online was introduced at ICI (now AstraZeneca) in 1984, and by 1988 was seen as one of the (if not the) most vital computer systems accessible by ICI's scientists (Warr & Haygarth-Jackson 1988).

Norman (1988) describes the principles of good design: that it should be obvious how something works (visibility); that there should be a distinct function for every control, and vice versa (mapping); that every action should have some associated feedback signal (and no delayed response); that there should be in-built constraints, to reduce the number of possible actions. Lastly, one should design to cater for errors, as to err is human; and one should minimize the amount of knowledge someone needs to retain (see Box 15.1).

Characteristics of those who choose to use these end-user systems

Although findings are somewhat contradictory (Nicholas & Harmarn 1985), they tend to fall into the following categories:

- those who are already active users of manual and hardcopy services (Haines 1982)
- those who have limited access to hard-copy sources, limited time, and good access to electronic sources (Nicholas & Harmarn 1985).

Conversely, it has been reported that those who trust the competence of information specialists tend to make less use of these systems (Bell 1990), although these findings are contradicted by others (Carey 1987, Jahoda & Bayer 1987).

Also, in environments where end-user searching does not persist beyond preliminary training, there is a trend towards the development of new, non-information scientist intermediaries (Mischo & Lee 1987).

Box 15.1
Application design:
impact on training

- Visibility
  —how something works is obvious from the design
  —standard interface eases learning
  —people will expect certain features from previous experience
- Mapping: e.g. one control button performs one function
- Feedback (immediate): on outcome of an action
- Knowledge in the world: versus in the head, i.e. minimizing what an individual needs to remember
- Constraints
  —to reduce the number of possible actions
  —sophisticated tools for expert users
  —complexity clutters learning for more basic users
- Design for error
  —to err is human
  —consequences of a mistake should not be disastrous
  —software itself acts as a training tool
  —error messages should be informative

Education and training of end-users

One of the main factors to ensure the success of end-user searching is availability of training (Cheney et al 1986). Continued, proactive training and support are also needed (Dedert & Johnson 1990). However, success is most likely where trainees make their own decision to acquire the necessary skills (Buntrock & Valicenti 1985a). Users also prefer to learn as they go by means of online help, or trial and error, and the ability to easily obtain assistance when needed (Mischo & Lee 1987). However, satisfaction is often higher for those who have had some form of formal training (classroom based or one-to-one—Igbaria & Nachman 1990). Training will be discussed more fully later in this chapter.

Operational constraints on end-users.

One of the major constraints is the availability or accessibility of hardware and software (Igbaria & Nachman 1990). Where these are easily available, end-users are most likely to use them. There are, however, a number of other potential barriers (Summitt 1989):

- getting started (or who do I call to get a password?)
- user interface design
- search failure
- perceived high cost
- overall lack of general awareness.

And also (Mischo & Lee 1987):

- other pressing demands on users' time
- convenience of using intermediaries

and (Guynes 1988, Tilson & East 1994)

- network problems and/or problems with connections.

Are end-users less motivated to do their own searching?

Demotivating factors are listed above. Also, users may be negatively influenced by anxiety, culture, age (Igbaria & Nachman 1990).

Reasons for motivation have been reported as convenience, speed (Sewell & Teitelbaum 1986), ability to browse (Faibisoff & Hurych 1981), confidence based on use of other computer systems (Haygarth-Jackson 1989), and expectations from previous experience in other organizations.

Will the end-user use the facility often enough to gain expertise?

The general consensus to this question would seem to be 'no' but does it matter (Faibisoff & Hurych 1981, McKibbon et al 1990)? For instance the user could use alternative means to supplement the information found, including asking an information specialist (Sewell & Teitelbaum 1986). This is generally recommended for comprehensive scientific or legal searches (Burris & Molinek 1991).

By and large, users are more interested in ease of use, and not concerned about exploiting the power of the search software (Tilson & East 1994).

Our main concern should be in the context of 'satisfied but inept' users—who do not realize what they might be missing (Scott 1989).

As with the findings of Ghilhardi 1996, mentioned at the beginning of this chapter, practitioners quote instances of decreases in some types of searches requested of information specialists, and increases in others (Salisbury et al 1990). A 1993 survey of 990 librarians in the US showed that end-user searching increased library activities by more than 30%, with an increase in complex searches and a broadening of the client base (Fisher & Bjorner 1994).

Practitioners also note the benefit derived in improved communication between end-users and information staff.

Will the end-user use the system often enough to make it cost-effective?

Referring back to Chapter 10, on the value and impact of information management, this is probably the wrong question to ask. What is more important is the more indirect, and harder to measure impact on the organization's productivity (Koenig 1990).

User-friendly systems

In the previous section, one of the main points under discussion was whether a system can be designed for use by the general end-user population. The example illustrated was end-user searching of CAS online databases, and how this came to be used extensively within an R&D environment. Now we are progressing to a new generation of end-user desktop tools which, incorporating the principles of good application design, have become more intuitive and generally require less training on the part of the end-user. This is exemplified in SciFinder from Chemical Abstracts Service (CAS), a research tool designed to assist scientists and researchers in locating information on a wide variety of chemistry-related topics.

Main features of SciFinder

SciFinder provides access to CAS databases, with more than 24 million substance records and over 16 million journal articles, patents and other documents. The application features interactive point and click methodology for retrieving information. The interface has a graphical basis, with the first screen that the user encounters offering buttons that are clearly defined for the major tasks that the end-user would wish to carry out (Fig 15.1).

The need for a complicated interface is minimized through the use of a hierarchical approach for user actions. This means that users are not confused and overwhelmed by initially being presented with all the possible search types. It is only by choosing the 'Explore'

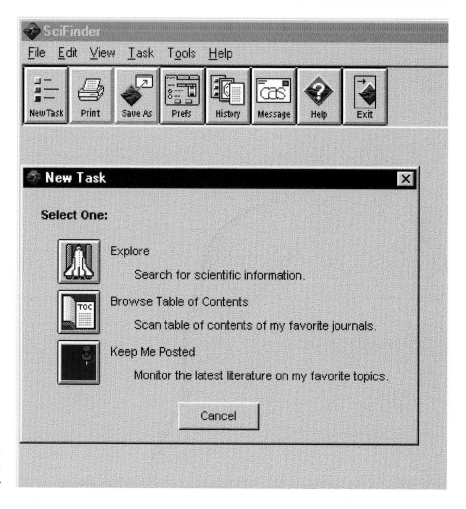

Figure 15.1 *Main search screen within SciFinder*

option that the user is presented with a further listing of search options. These options include the expected actions of chemical substance and reaction searching, with the additional choices of research topic, author and information retrieval via a specific reference, e.g. CA accession number (Fig. 15.2).

Although many types of search are possible within SciFinder, the 'Explore by Research Topic' is perhaps one that best illustrates the requirements of a user-friendly system and it will be this search feature that will be discussed here.

Use of the 'Explore by Research Topic' feature in SciFinder

To enter a query in 'Explore by Research Topic', the user simply has to type words or phrases pertaining to the research topic in exactly the same way as they would say or write them. SciFinder's intelligent natural language search algorithm negates the need for the user to enter queries using conventional Boolean search logic. SciFinder determines the keywords and combines them in a logical manner. The user can also use negative terms to describe a search topic with the inclusion of terms such as 'NOT' and 'EXCEPT', thus providing flexibility in query formulation. SciFinder can also recognize commonly used abbreviations and also will allow for misspelling and US/British English differences such as 'colour' and 'color'.

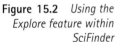

Figure 15.2 *Using the Explore feature within SciFinder*

An example search is shown in Figure 15.3.

When an 'Explore by Research Topic' search is carried out, initially the user is presented with a breakdown of the clustering of references matching the search criteria (Fig. 15.4).

By choosing the first option, those references where the search terms have been found to be closely associated with one another can be retrieved. Scanning the titles of results returned, one can see the effect of smart searching within SciFinder, as the fifth paper listed has the keyword 'patients' highlighted, indicating that the search algorithm has expanded 'humans' to also include 'patients' (Fig. 15.5). To see the abstract details for a particular record, the user can click on the microscope icon in the title display screen.

SciFinder offers the user the capability to further analyse the result sets, via a number of predefined criteria (Fig. 15.6), such as author name or company/organization.

Of particular usefulness is the 'Analyse by Company/Organization' option, which presents the search results grouped by company/organization. The results are shown in a histogram format, which allows the user easily to see which organization is most active in the research area of interest. This is illustrated in Figure 15.7, where the results of the previous search have been analysed and it can be seen that Nihon University, Japan has 19 references in the area of 'Hepatitis C and humans'. Thus the user can easily answer a question that in other systems would involve many more steps and detailed post-search analysis.

User-friendly systems—the future

As applications become more intuitive, the natural progression will be to provide a seamless integration between primary and secondary literature sources. The user will want to make use of intelligent search capabilities, whilst being able to link easily to the original

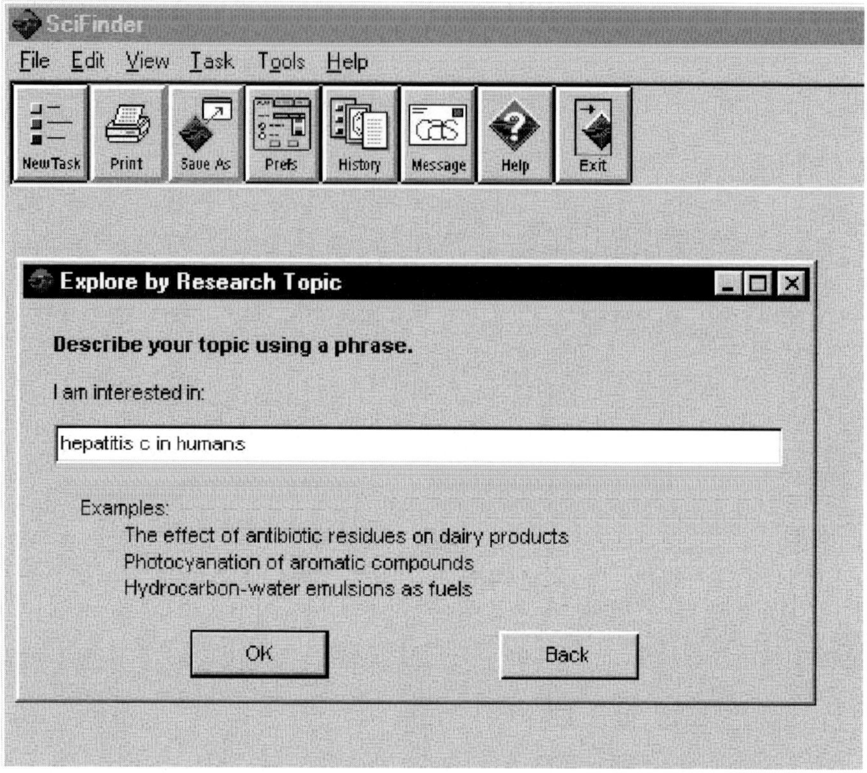

Figure 15.3 *Explore by Research Topic*

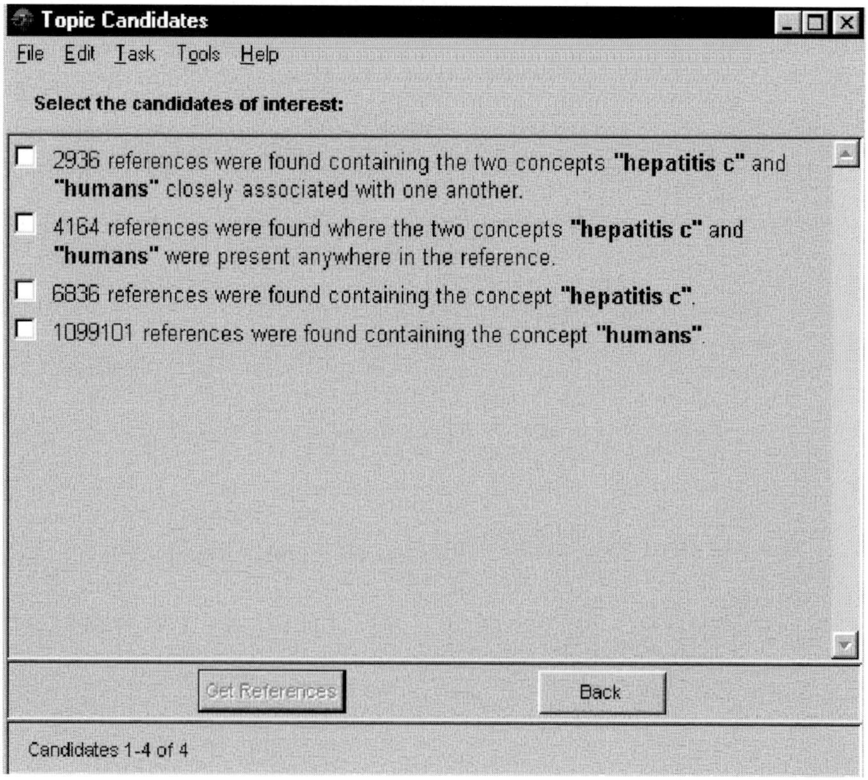

Figure 15.4
Presentation of initial results from Explore by Research Topic

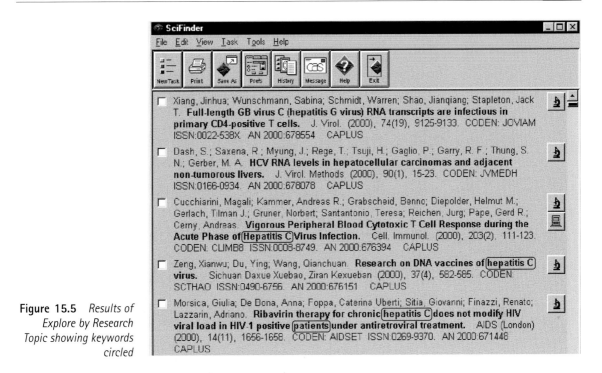

article. Progress towards this ideal situation is being made, and the most recent release of
SciFinder (v5.0) allows the user to carry out a search and, subject to licence agreements with
major journal publishers, to link to the article level through use of the ChemPort connection.
Future developments with SciFinder will extend these capabilities with the addition of links
to citation information, the ability to explore by company/organization name and the development of data visualization.

The role of the information professional in supporting the end-user

The changing role of intermediaries

Traditional definitions of information specialists, information scientists or special librarians focus on their role as intermediaries. In the early 1980s their role, particularly in the
pharmaceutical industry R&D environment, was seen as receiving end-user queries and
translating them into the language of the appropriate information source, usually computer-based bibliographic database(s) and host systems (Box 15.2). They provided the
end-user with the result of the search, usually after some prior evaluation of the information (Tilson & East 1994). Intermediaries would not normally anticipate the search,
they would respond to a specific request from the end-user. To this 'reactive' role was
added the 'proactive' current awareness role described elsewhere in this book. Fisher and
Bjorner (1994) described the role of some information specialists as that of an internal
consultant (Box 15.2).

Nick Moore (1996) elegantly captures these various roles when he describes how technology is influencing the way information is used, as well as the way in which information professionals work. In 1996 he believed that we would see the emergence of three
complementary groups of information professionals.

Box 15.2 *The changing role of the information specialist*

1980. The intermediary:

■ Provides search services: receives end user queries; translates them into language of appropriate information source, often computerized; provides results of the search, possibly after prior evaluation

■ Provides current awareness services: achieved by matching awareness of end-user needs with sources of information available; possibly in electronic form

1994. The internal consultant:

■ Recommends appropriate sources

■ Educates departmental information 'gatekeepers'

■ Trains end-users

■ Integrates internal and external information

■ Selects the right medium/approach for managing information (e.g. in databases)

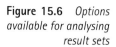

Figure 15.6 *Options available for analysing result sets*

Creators

They are information professionals who will develop and produce information products and services. They will need skills in information and how it works; in navigation to help people find their way around a 'system'; in design (layout, typography and general design

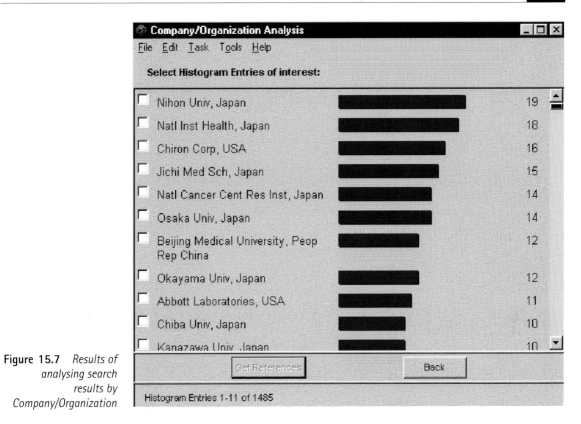

Figure 15.7 *Results of analysing search results by Company/Organization*

principles). Through their work 'it should be as easy to switch from using one information system to another as it is to switch from driving one car to another.'

Communicators (or consultants)

'Information comes best when wrapped in a person.' Communicators will tailor the information provided by computer-based systems to an individual's needs. They will need strong interpersonal skills to adapt to the individual's characteristics; analytical skills to distinguish between actual needs and expressed demands, and to analyse and select the information available. They will also need to make good use of information resources and tools to find/retrieve information. Many will also need a high level of subject knowledge.

Consolidators

Decision-support systems and executive information systems alone are not enough as they require managers to spend significant amounts of time in order to find the information they need. A consolidator will collect information from a wide range of sources, analyse it and synthesize it to provide a rich, complete, yet easy to digest picture of the subject in which a manager is interested. Consolidators will thus reduce the burden on managers. As well as the above skills, they will need to be able to see patterns and make connections, present the results effectively (in writing or verbally), and to reduce complexity without sacrificing accuracy.

David Bawden of City University London (unpublished communications) argues that a range of roles has always been present, but that it is the balance, or emphasis on these which changes with changes in technology. Thus there are the:

1. custodian—who is responsible for maintaining quality and access to information
2. producer—who generates information
3. compiler—who will pull together information from various sources
4. evaluator
5. interpreter/analyst—who will take information and process it in some way to aid understanding or assimilation by the intended audience
6. educator/trainer
7. consultant/evangelist—who will encourage the use of information by others.

Roles 4, 6, 7 are particularly important at the moment. The educator/trainer is concerned with the effective use of information systems to meet individuals' needs. The consultant provides guidance in the wise use of information resources, to minimize information overload. The evaluator advises on the value of the content of alternative sources. The evangelist promotes the use of information resources.

Education/training and support

Training programmes for end-user applications need to be introduced within the context and time-frame of overall project management for implementing new systems. Too often the focus of such projects is on the technological solution, and training is addressed as a final add-on, together with any plans for marketing and supporting the application (Goodman 1998).

Indeed, many would argue that the ideal is not to need any formal method of training at all, but instead the interface to the application should be so intuitive that learning to use it is as simple as changing from one car to another once proficiency in driving has been achieved. Many designers and/or implementers of new applications erroneously assume that users are already proficient.

I would like to share three key insights with readers:

- that the planning for training needs to start in the early stages of a project tasked with the implementation of a new end-user application
- that marketing, training and support are a continuum of activities, all geared to optimizing the effective use of end-user systems
- that designers of applications need to be continuously attuned to the need for minimizing the need for formal training.

Orna (1990) states that 'whenever change is contemplated, the consequences for the whole socio-technical system need to be carefully considered from the start and taken into account in the specification for any new technical systems'. The 'socio-technical' approach considers how people think, work, do their tasks and interact when using technology.

Box 15.3 *Some definitions*

Marketing/Communication
a series of messages given to customers so that they understand the reason for the introduction of a new end-user product, the benefits, and when/how they will be affected by it

Training—knowledge transfer
the major activity by which customers learn the new skills necessary to use new products and embed their use into their way of working

Support
the materials and organizational structures needed to help customers use the new product successfully once initial training is completed

Planning training and associated activities (Goodman 1998)

Preparations for communication, training and support rely on a good understanding of:

1. The target audience(s), and of how the new application will be used and affect their environments (the 'change event'). It is necessary to do a fair amount of research to gain this understanding. Many approaches are possible, from looking at logs of usage of previous similar or related systems, to user surveys, interviews, focus groups and pilots. Carefully planned pilots will be invaluable for gathering or consolidating such information, as well as for testing out training/support approaches for eventual implementation.

2. The literature abounds in market research/analysis techniques which can be useful at this stage of the exercise. The 4 Ps, the 4 Cs and SWOT analysis are some examples of these. The 4 Ps are: Product, Place, Promotion, Price (Condous 1983). In a service environment, service should be added. The 4 Cs are: Convenience, Cost to the user, Communication, Customer needs and wants (Webber 1995). SWOT stands for: Strengths, Weaknesses, Opportunities, Threats. A SWOT analysis can be used to understand the end-user's perspective of an application and how training should be targeted to address this.

3. Having established the target audience(s) and how the new application will affect their business processes, it will be necessary to carry out some form of training needs analysis. This is essentially a form of gap analysis. What type and level of behaviour, understanding or knowledge and skills do you want to achieve as the result of training? Where are your audience now with respect to those targets? What is the gap to be bridged? The trend is to take a task-based approach in this analysis, i.e. make the training relevant to the activities which the customer needs to perform, rather than covering all the details of how an application works.

4. The training needs will in turn help to establish the learning objectives. From the objectives you can begin to define the content material to meet these objectives. As with all objectives, these need to be SMART – Specific, Measurable, Achievable, Relevant (to the customers), and Time-scaled.

Once this ground work has been done, the approaches to be used for delivering the communication, training and support can be selected. A range of approaches may be needed to meet individuals' preferred methods of learning (see Box 15.4). One-to-one approaches

---

Box 15.4 *Training and support*

Criteria for selecting alternative approaches
- Training/support staff interest, ability, experience
- Size of intended audience
- Time available to trainers and audience
- Nature/level of instruction planned
- Requirements for and availability of equipment/facilities
- Times/costs involved in revising materials for continued use

Alternative approaches

Lectures or presentations and demonstrations	User meetings, 'brown bag' lunches, seminars
Formal course (targeted or general)	Desk-side training, clinics (or workshops)
Programmed instruction: computer-assisted module or workbook	Training videos, cassettes, other audiovisual
Information sheets or reference guides (e.g. 'Tipsheets', Q&A, FAQs)	Online help

are the most effective means of getting complex messages and instruction across to end-users. Electronic communications, computer-based tutorials and online help, or large auditorium presentations with demonstrations are effective ways of reaching a large audience with minimum resources involved in delivery. The trend is to use customized computer-based tutorials, online help and electronic forms of one-to-one assistance (Meadow et al 1994).

Freeman et al (1995) provide access to external databases through networked CD-ROMs. They have included a computer-based tutorial on the front-end (complemented with a paper-based workbook) to help users develop search strategies and skills. Conversely BIDS (Bath Information & Data Services), used by students at UK universities to access a range of information sources via the web, rely on a user group and a range of hard-copy publicity and training materials (Morrow 1995).

Fisher & Bjorner (1994) recommend that an individual's learning should involve a number of training sessions over time and not just rely on a one-off classroom course. Additionally they, as do Meadow et al (1994), emphasize the need to extend training from a focus on search strategies and the mechanics of using various databases and technologies, to the broader context of information literacy. In this context, 'information literacy' means that users can formalize their requirements, are able to identify appropriate sources, use them effectively, and organize, evaluate and use the resultant information. Dedert and Johnson (1990) trained end-users to search databases on the STN host system. They found that the most effective method was a short (one-and-a-half hour) training session, accompanied by individual 30–minute practice sessions supplemented by the availability of tutorial disks, a booklet and the option of a novice mode of searching.

Preparing training materials

Having completed the planning, the next step is the more detailed design and preparation of the training material. There are a number of authoritative books on 'instructional design' (Reay 1994, Kemp et al 1994). A decision will have to be taken on the most appropriate methods of training: instructor-led classes, training manuals, or computer-based training (CBT) and internets or intranets (IBT or WBT). The various forms of computer-based training are the most complex because they have the flexibility of using a range of simulations and interactive programmes. They can also allow for different learning paths based on the needs of the users. However, production of CBTs requires skills in graphic design, installation etc.

Evaluating the training

It is obviously important to get user input and feedback when first preparing the training programme, and when implementing it. Ideally, the programme should be piloted with a sample of users before implementation. Again, there are a number of authoritative books in this area (Reay 1994, Kemp et al 1994). It is important when evaluating training during or after implementation to understand the difference between assessing whether, and how well, the original objectives of the training have been met, and assessing how well the training is actually translated in the workplace. Different evaluation approaches will yield these different types of information which in turn need to be fed back, iteratively, into the planning programme.

Implementation

Effective delivery of training requires its own set of skills, especially if instructor-led training is chosen. It is important to recognize this fact at the planning stage, and consider whether to use the organization's own internal staff, or whether to bring in specialized trainers.

Tools for end-user support.

A wide range of tools is available for end-user support (see Fig. 15.8).

Job aids or reference tools

Rosset & Gautier-Downes (1991) provide a very useful overview of these mechanisms, which they describe as 'job aids'. They define a job aid as 'a repository for information, processes or perspectives that is external to the individual, and that supports work and activity by directing, guiding and enlightening performance'. They differentiate between instruction, which 'usually happens before a need arises and builds the capacity of the individual', and job aids which 'act as references whenever the need to know arises'.

A good way to introduce job aids is to use them in the course of instruction so that end-users become used to referring to them when they need to. Job aids are usually used during performance of a task, but could also be used beforehand to prepare, or afterwards to review the task. Expert systems, performance support tools and online help are examples of job aids for coaching, advising and supporting the user.

Support by colleagues and/or help desk

While many organizations have help desks to support end-users, they vary in the organizational location of these help desks, and the degree of involvement by information staff or even end-users themselves. End-user involvement in the support of their colleagues may be more or less formal.

Duncan & Guthrie (1995) presented a very entertaining and informative case study of how they recruited and trained 50 end-users to act as the first line of support for 750 staff at the Florida Lottery. Being the land of Disneyworld they used a magic and adventure theme throughout to create enthusiasm and commitment for this approach—but the whole programme was soundly underwritten with clear contracts of commitment from these help desk 'wizards', their managers and the help desk itself. Their method for persuading managers to have staff take on what is still an informal role (it is not written into their job descriptions) included the following:

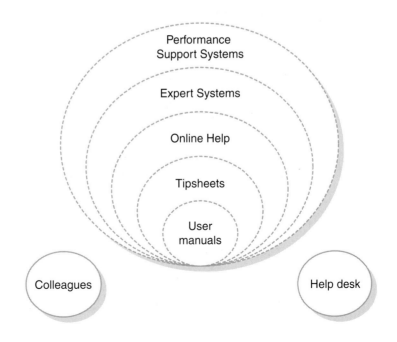

Figure 15.8
Mechanisms for providing end-user support

■ An assessment of how many additional help desk staff would be needed to support their range of applications: they calculated a need for 50–60 additional staff, asked for five and were turned down!

■ Identification of end-users who were already providing this kind of informal support: they argued that by giving them formal training, and having all commit to taking only 5% of their time for the new arrangement, they would be ensuring that the support given would be more effective, and make less use of their time than previously

Conclusion

How to help end-users make effective use of information resources continues to be a major issue in the pharmaceutical industry, health services and other organizations. Those of us who provide information services need to be aware of this, and develop strategies and programmes to guide our customers in deciding when to use desktop tools, and when to seek assistance from information professionals. We need to be able to influence the design of desktop tools for optimum use by end-users, and we must continue to develop our skills as coaches, consultants and users of these resources ourselves.

References and further Reading

Bell G 1990 Online searching in industry versus academia: a study in partnerships. Online September: 15–56

Bennett J L 1970 Interactive bibliographic search as a challenge to interface design. IBM Research September Report no. RJ755

Buntrock R E, Valicenti A K 1985a End-users and chemical information. Journal of Chemical Information and Computer Science 25(3): 203–207

Buntrock R E, Valicenti A K 1985b End-user searching: the Amoco experience. Journal of Chemical Information and Computer Science 25(4): 415–419

Burris R A, Molinek F R 1991 Establishing and managing a successful end-user search service in a large special library. Online March: 36–39

Carey K 1987 Online searching: making the switch from an academic to a corporate environment. Proceedings of the 1987 Online Meeting: 53–56

Cheney P H, Mann R I, Amoroso D L 1986 Organisational factors affecting the success of end-user computing. Journal of Management Information Systems 3(1): 65–80

Condous C 1983 Non-profit marketing—libraries' future? Aslib Proceedings 35(10): 407–417

Cornick D 1989 Being an end-user is not for everyone. Online March: 49–54

Dedert P L, Johnson D K 1990 Promoting and supporting end-user online searching in an industrial research environment: a survey of experiences at Exxon Research Engineering Company. Science and Technology Libraries 10(1): 25–46

Duncan C, Guthrie S 1995 Paper presented at Computing Training and Support Orlando, Oct 1st-4th

Duplessis J P, Vanbiljon J A, Tolmie C J, et al 1995 A model for intelligent computer-aided education systems. Computers and Education 24: 89–106

Eisenberg M 1983 The direct use of online bibliographic information systems by untrained end-users: a review of research. ERIC Clearinghouse on Information Resources NY, Syracuse, NY

Erkkila J E 1990 CD-ROM vs online: implications for management from the cost side. Canadian Library Journal 47(6): 421–428

Faibisoff S G, Hurych J 1981 Is there a future for the end-user in online bibliographis searching? Special Libraries 72(4): 347–355

Fisher J, Bjorner S 1994 Enabling online end-user searching: an expanding role for librarians. Special Libraries Fall: 281–291

Freeman H, Rouse R, Hilton A 1995 Making the most of electronic databases. Computer-bases tutorials for a CD-ROM network. Managing Information 2(1/2): 36–38

Ghilhardi F J M 1996 End-users: they come and grow. Searcher June: 55–56

Goodman E 1998 A methodology for the 'use-sensitive implementation' of information systems in the pharmaceutical industry: a case study. International Journal of Information Management 18(2): 121–138

Guyes J L 1988 Impact of system response time on state anxiety. Communications of the ACM 31(3): 342–347

Haines J S 1982 Experiences in training end-user searchers. Online November: 14–23

Haygarth-Jackson A 1989 Conclusions and the future. In: Cronin B (ed) Foundations of information science, vol 4: training and education for online. IIS/Taylor Graham, pp 223–225

Igbaria M, Nachman S A 1990 Correlates of user satisfaction with end-user computing: an exploratory study. Information and Management 19(2): 73–82

Jahoda G, Bayer A E 1987 Online searches: characteristics of users and uses in one academic and one industrial organization. Proceedings of the ASIS Annual Meeting: 165–167

Kemp J E, Morrison G R, Ross S M 1994 Designing effective instruction. Macmillan College Publishing, Basingstoke

Koenig M E D 1990 The information and library environment and the productivity of research. Paper presented at the International Federation of Library Associations 56th General Conference, Stockholm, Sweden

Kolb D 1981 Learning styles and disciplinary differences. In: The modern American college. Jossey-Bass, San Fransisco: AW Chickering and Associates pp 232–255

McKibbon K A, Haynes R B, Walker-Dilks J M et al 1994 How good are clinical Medline searches? A comparative study of clinical end-user and librarian searches. Computers and Biomedical Research 23(6): 583–593

Marshall J G, Allen S 1990 Training and assistance techniques for database users. Canadian Journal of Information Science 15(2): 38–49

Meadow C T 1979 Online searching and computer programming. Some behavioural similarities (or . . . why end-users will eventually take over the terminal). Online 3(1): 49–52

Meadow C T, Marchionini G, Cherry J M 1994 Speculations on the measurement and use of user characteristics in information retrieval experimentation. Canadian Journal of Information and Library Science 19: 1–22

Mischo W H, Lee J 1987 End-user searching of bibliographic databases. ARIST 22 ch. 7: 227–263

Moore N 1996 Creators, communicators, consolidators: the new information professional. Managing Information 3(6): 24–25

Morrow T 1995 BIDS—the growth of a network end-user bibliographic database service. Program 29(1): 31–41

Nicholas D, Harman J 1985 The end-user: an assessment and review of the literature. Social Science Studies 5(4): 173–184

Norman D A 1988 The psychology of everyday things. Basic Books, New York

Orna E 1990 Practical information policies. How to manage information flow in organisations. Gower, Aldershot

Reay D G 1994 Understanding how people learn. Kogan Page, London

Rae L 1994 The trainer development programme. 10-day training programme of workshop sessions. Kogan Page, London

Ring G 1994 Electronic performance support systems in higher education. In: Beattie K, McNaught C, Wills S (eds) Interactive multimedia in university education: designing for change in teaching and learning. IFIP: Elsevier Science, pp 193–203

Rossett A, Gautier-Downs J 1991 A handbook of job aids. Pfeiffer & Company, San Diego

Salisbury L, Toombs H S, Kelly E A, et al 1990 The effect of end-user searching on reference services: experience with Medline and Current Contents. Bulletin of the Medical Library Association 78(2): 188–191

Schilling K, Ginn D S, Mickelson P, et al 1995 Integration of information-seeking skills and activities into problem-based curriculum. Bulletin of the Medical Library Association 83: 176–183

Scott T 1989 On the satisfied and inept end-user. Medical Reference Quarterly 8(1): 45–48

Sewell W, Teitelbaum S 1986 Observations of end-user online searching behaviour over eleven years. Journal of the American Society for Information Science 37(4): 243–245

Summitt R K 1989 In search of the elusive end-user. Online Review 13(6): 485–491

Tilson Y, East H 1994 Academic scientists' reaction to end-user services: observations on a trial service giving access to Medline using the Grateful Med software. Online and CD-ROM Review 18(2): 71–77

Ting-Ming L 1988 The evaluation of end-user online searching: a review of the literature. Journal of Library and Information Science (USA/Taiwan) 14(1): 62–84

Walker G 1988 End-user searching: a selection of the literature for 1983–1988. ERIC Clearinghouse on Information Resources, Syracuse, NY

Warr W A R, Haygarth-Jackson A R 1988 End-user searching of CAS Online. Results of a cooperative experiment between Imperial Chemical Industries and Chemical Abstracts Service. Journal of Chemical Information and Computer Science 28: 68–72

Webber S 1995 Marketing library information services. Inform 173: 5

White T 1995 Realising the vision. End-user training and support. IT Training February/March: 17–23

Whittall S J 1988 End-user searching with CD-ROM. Proceedings of the 15th Annual Conference AIOPI: 122–135

Witiak J 1988 What is the role of the intermediary in end-user training? Online September: 50–52

Chapter 16

Codes of practice for the pharmaceutical industry

Heather Simmonds

Introduction

Information departments both within and outside the pharmaceutical industry need to understand and be aware of the requirements of the law and codes of practice in relation to the preparation of promotional material for medicines. Assessing such material is an important aspect of the work of both pharmaceutical industry information departments and drug information pharmacists.

The role of medical information departments in pharmaceutical companies is to provide technical support for the company's activities. One of the major activities is to provide detailed assistance in relation to the promotion of medicines. Companies devote enormous resources to ensuring that medicines are promoted in accordance with statutory and other requirements. The commitment of the pharmaceutical industry to providing high quality effective medicines brings major benefits to health and the economy. Investment into researching and developing medicines in the UK amounts to over £7 million per day, with each medicine costing approximately £350 million and taking an average of 10–12 years to develop before it is authorized for use. The pharmaceutical industry therefore considers it vital to keep health professionals and the public informed about its products and to promote their rational use.

Codes of practice in the UK and statutory requirements

In relation to the promotion of medicines in the UK, the Code of Practice for the Pharmaceutical Industry was established by the Association of the British Pharmaceutical Industry (ABPI) in 1958 to set standards for the promotion of medicines to the health professions. It has been regularly updated since then. This chapter refers to the edition of the Code that came into operation on 1 January 1998 (PMCPA 1998).

The Code applies to the promotion of medicines to members of the UK health professions and to appropriate administrative staff and to information made available to the public about medicines so promoted. The ABPI Code does not apply to the promotion of over-the-counter medicines to members of the health professions when the object is to encourage purchase by members of the general public, nor does it apply to advertisements for over-the-counter medicines to the general public for self-medication purposes. These advertisements are covered by two codes established by the Proprietary Association of Great Britain.

Legal requirements in the UK were first introduced under the provisions of the Medicines Act (1968) and in 1978 the first detailed regulations controlling the promotion of medicines were made. In 1992 European Council Directive 92/28/EEC (EEC 1992) on the advertising of medicinal products for human use was adopted. This set out the requirements for members of the European Union and was implemented in the UK by The Medicines (Advertising) Regulations (1994—amended 1996) and The Medicines (Monitoring of Advertising) Regulations (1994—amended 1999). All of the codes reflect the legal requirements with some extending beyond the legal requirements.

ABPI Code of Practice for the Pharmaceutical Industry

This section will cover in detail the promotion of medicines to healthcare professionals for prescribing and the ABPI Code of Practice for the Pharmaceutical Industry (PMCPA 1998).

There have been many changes since the first version of the Code. Originally the Code dealt primarily with promotion to doctors and dentists but since 1993 it has covered promotion to members of the health professions in general and to appropriate administrative staff such as, for example, hospital managers. Promotion is defined as any activity undertaken by a pharmaceutical company or with its authority which promotes the prescription, supply, sale or administration of its medicines. The Code covers journal and direct mail advertising, the activities of representatives, including materials used by representatives, the supply of samples, the provision of inducements, the provision of hospitality, the sponsorship of meetings, the provision of information to the general public and all other sales promotion in whatever form, including promotion on the internet. The principles of the Code apply whatever the method of communication.

The aim of the Code is to ensure that the promotion of medicines to members of the health professions and to administrative staff is carried out in a responsible, ethical and professional manner. Strong support is given to the Code by the industry, with pharmaceutical companies devoting considerable resources to ensure that their promotional activities comply with the Code.

Establishment of the Authority

The Prescription Medicines Code of Practice Authority (PMCPA) was established by the ABPI in 1993 to operate the Code independently of the ABPI itself. The Constitution and Procedure for the Code of Practice Authority appears at the back of the Code of Practice booklet (PMCPA 1998).

Compliance with the Code is obligatory for ABPI member companies and in addition some 70 or so non-member companies have voluntarily agreed to comply with the Code and to accept the jurisdiction of the Authority.

Companies are responsible for ensuring that their promotional activities comply with the Code. Details of the complaint procedure are given in the Code of Practice booklet. To summarize, each complaint is considered by the Code of Practice Panel, which consists of the three members of the Code of Practice Authority acting with the assistance of expert advice where appropriate. The decisions of the Panel can be appealed by the parties to the Code of Practice Appeal Board. The Appeal Board is chaired by an independent, legally qualified chairman and includes three medically qualified independent members, an independent pharmacist and an independent member from a body which provides information on medicines. The remainder of the Appeal Board is comprised of eight senior executives and four medical directors of pharmaceutical companies. The Appeal Board is the final arbiter on complaints under the Code. The Appeal Board also oversees the work of the Panel and gives advice to the Authority as required.

Where a breach of the Code is ruled, the company concerned must give an undertaking that use of the material and/or the practice in question has ceased forthwith and that all possible steps have been taken to avoid a similar breach of the Code in the future. An undertaking must be accompanied by details of the action taken to implement the ruling. Additional sanctions are imposed in serious cases. Reports on all cases are published by the Authority in the quarterly Code of Practice Review. The Review is widely circulated and serves two purposes, first as a sanction when breaches of the Code are ruled and, second, for educational purposes.

Requirements of the Code of particular relevance

This section highlights the clauses of the Code which are particularly relevant to medical information departments. It is not exhaustive and information personnel should ensure that they are familiar with the Code in its entirety.

Clause 1.2 Definition of promotion

The definition of promotion does not include replies made in response to individual enquiries from members of the health professions or in reply to specific communications, including letters published in journals, if the replies relate solely to the subject matter of the enquiry, are accurate and do not mislead and are not promotional in nature. The response must be tailored to the enquiry. Information departments are often required to respond to such requests. Standard replies can be prepared but can be used only when they directly and solely relate to the particular enquiry. Documents must not have the appearance of promotional material.

Clause 3 Marketing authorization

A pharmaceutical company must not promote a medicine prior to the grant of its marketing authorization. Promotion must be in accordance with the marketing authorization and must not be inconsistent with the summary of product characteristics (SPC) or data sheet. The legitimate exchange of medical and scientific information during the development of a medicine is permitted provided that the information/activity does not constitute promotion. The supplementary information to Clause 3 refers to advance notification of new products or product changes which have significant budgetary implications. This is an exemption for the supply of limited information to persons responsible for making policy decisions on budgets rather than those expected to prescribe the product.

Medical/generic representatives might be asked about products in development or indications yet to be approved. It is not acceptable for representatives to initiate discussions with health professionals about unlicensed medicines or unauthorized indications. Such enquiries are best dealt with by the medical information department.

Clause 7 Information, claims and comparisons

The majority of cases fall under the requirements of Clause 7 and the principles of the Code are probably best summed up in Clauses 7.2 and 7.3. Clause 7.2 requires that information, claims and comparisons must be accurate, balanced, fair, objective and unambiguous and must be based on an up-to-date evaluation of all the evidence and reflect that evidence clearly. They must not mislead either directly or by implication. Clause 7.3 requires that any information, claim or comparison must be capable of substantiation and substantiation must be provided without delay to members of the health professions or appropriate administrative staff upon request. Requests for such substantiation often come from health professionals in competitor companies. The ABPI encourages companies to discuss matters together prior to bringing complaints to the Authority and often there is a large amount of correspondence between companies prior to complaints being made. Inter-company activity represents a powerful component in the success of self-regulation as competing companies carefully scrutinize each other's promotional material and frequently ask for supporting evidence. It is often a useful exercise when drawing up or approving promotional material to consider what would be sent in response to a request for substantiation. It cannot be pleaded when such a request is received that the evidence is confidential or otherwise unavailable. The preparation of promotional material is an important task and a number of pharmaceutical companies use the expertise of information personnel, particularly medical information departments, in the development of promotional materials. Medical information staff may identify supporting references as well as assess the claims etc. to ensure compliance with the Code.

Clause 9 Format, suitability and causing offence, sponsorship

All materials and activities must recognize the special nature of medicines and the professional standing of the audience and must not be likely to cause offence. High standards must be maintained at all times. Telephone, email and facsimile must not be used for promotional purposes except with the prior permission of the recipient.

Clause 9.9 of the Code requires that material relating to medicines and their uses which is sponsored by a pharmaceutical company must clearly indicate such sponsorship. The declaration of sponsorship must be sufficiently prominent to ensure that readers are aware of it at the outset. Any treatment guidelines sponsored by a pharmaceutical company must be reasonable and reflect the opinion of the majority of experts in the field.

Clause 10 Disguised promotion

Promotional material and activity must not be disguised. Companies must be careful to be open and up-front about the origin of documents and guidelines etc. Genuine guidelines developed by an independent group are often circulated by a pharmaceutical company. The involvement of the company in such activities must, however, be made entirely clear.

Non-promotional items such as independently produced guidelines can become subject to the Code simply because of the way that companies have used such items, for example by handing them on to doctors etc.

Research activities, post-marketing surveillance studies, clinical assessments and the like must not be disguised promotion.

Clause 13 Scientific service responsible for information

Companies must have a scientific service to compile and collate all information, whether received from medical representatives or from any other source about the medicines which they market. The scientific service is usually the medical information department.

Clause 14 Certification of promotional material

Medical information personnel are often involved in their company's approval system. Occasionally they are appointed as signatories, but more usually medical information departments are involved prior to final sign-off, acting as an important check. No promotional material can be issued unless its final form has been certified by two people on behalf of the company. One must be medically qualified and the other must be an appropriately qualified person or a senior official of the company. The names and qualifications have to be notified in advance to the Medicines Control Agency (MCA) and the Authority.

The signatories sign a certificate to say that they have examined the material in its final form and that it is in accordance with the relevant advertising regulations and the Code, is not inconsistent with the SPC and is a fair and truthful presentation of the facts about the medicine.

Guidelines on company procedures relating to the Code are included at the back of the Code of Practice booklet and information personnel should be familiar with them. The guidelines provide advice about many of the Code's requirements. In relation to certification, the guidelines point out that each certificate should bear a reference number, with the same number appearing on the advertisement. Different sizes and layouts should be separately certified.

Clause 15 Representatives

Medical information departments have regular contact with representatives, frequently responding to enquiries from them. Some medical information departments are involved in training representatives as well as general training on the Code for other staff. Materials used to train representatives must comply with the Code. The Code applies to what representatives say as well as what they do. Representatives must pass the appropriate ABPI examination within two years of commencing work as a representative.

Clause 20 Relations with the general public and the media

The introduction of patient pack information leaflets with medicines has contributed to the increased amount of information now available to the patient. Information departments often deal with requests from patients. Pharmaceutical companies can provide information to the public provided that it meets the requirements of Clause 20. European Directive 92/28/EEC, UK law and Clause 20.1 prohibit the advertising of prescription only medicines (POMs) to the general public. This restriction also applies to certain medicines which are not POM but which nonetheless cannot be legally advertised to the general public. Under the Code companies can, however, make information about medicines available to the public directly or indirectly provided that it meets certain criteria. These are set out under Clause 20.2. The information must be factual and presented in a balanced way. It must not raise unfounded hopes of successful treatment or be misleading with respect to the safety of the product. Statements must not be made for the purpose of encouraging members of the public to ask their doctors to prescribe a specific medicine. Companies are permitted to provide European Public Assessment Reports (EPARs) or SPCs to members of the public on request. Similarly, companies can provide copies of patient pack information leaflets to the public on request. The *ABPI Compendium of Data Sheets and Summaries of Product Characteristics* and the *ABPI Patient Information Leaflet Compendium* are available for purchase by the public and are in most reference libraries in the UK. Access is also available via the internet (www.emc.vhn.net). The supplementary information to Clause 20.2 allows for financial information to be made available to inform shareholders, the stock exchange and the like by way of annual reports and announcements etc.

There has been much discussion recently about the prohibition on advertising POMs to the public. Patients are demanding more information about medicines. No change can be made to the Code in this respect unless European Directive 92/28/EEC (EEC 1992) and UK law are first amended. The debate about this area has resulted in part from the increased availability of information via the internet. The internet has highlighted the differences between the United States of America, where the advertising of POMs to the public is permitted, and Europe, where such advertising is prohibited. The Authority has issued guidance about the use of the internet. The difficulties relate to the potential audience and jurisdiction and arise largely from the international nature of the internet. Pharmaceutical companies based in the UK must develop closed user groups if they wish to advertise POMs to healthcare professionals. Material on open access sites is available to the public and should therefore comply with Clause 20. SPCs, patient information leaflets and EPARs can be placed on open access sites by pharmaceutical companies.

Other codes

International

The International Federation of Pharmaceutical Manufacturers Associations (IFPMA) Code of Pharmaceutical Marketing Practices sets out minimum standards for the promotion of medicines to healthcare professionals. The Code, established in 1981, is intended to define universally applicable baseline standards of marketing practices and to provide an operational code to be used in countries other than those in which a more demanding national code operates. The IFPMA Code applies to any company belonging to at least one member association of the IFPMA in all the countries of the world where that company does business. Companies entering into licensing and agency agreements are expected to require their licensees and agents to respect the provisions of the IFPMA Code.

European

The European Federation of Pharmaceutical Industries' Associations (EFPIA) Code of Practice for the Promotion of Medicines (1992) applies to all members of EFPIA. The Code was introduced in 1991 during the development of what became the Council directive on the advertising of medicinal products for human use. EFPIA does not deal with complaints—they are referred to the local trade association. EFPIA prepares an report each year.

The ABPI Code incorporates the IFPMA and EFPIA Codes insofar as they are not incompatible with UK Law.

Conclusion

Information departments play important roles in the production and assessment of promotional material as well as providing advice.

One of the Authority's roles is to provide informal advice and guidance on the application of the Code. Information personnel should not hesitate to contact the Authority if they are in doubt as to the interpretation of the Code.

References and Further Reading

Association of the British Pharmaceutical Industry, The (ABPI) 2000 Compendium of data sheets and summaries of product characteristics. Datapharm, Epsom (Datapharm Publications Limited, Novellus Court, 61 South Street, Epsom, Surrey, KT18 7PX)

Association of the British Pharmaceutical Industry, The (ABPI) 1995 Patient information leaflet compendium. Datapharm, Epsom

European Economic Community (EEC) 1992 European Council Directive 92/28/EEC.

European Federation of Pharmaceutical Industries' Association (EFPIA) 1992 European code of practice for the promotion of medicines. EFPIA, Brussels (EFPIA, Rue du Trône 108, 1050, Brussels, Belgium. Telephone 00 322 626 2555)

International Federation of Pharmaceutical Manufacturers Associations (IFPMA) 1994 Code of pharmaceutical marketing practices. IFPMA, Geneva (IFPMA, 30 Rue de St Jean, 1211 Geneva 18, Switzerland. Telephone 004122 340 1200) www.ifpma.org

Medicines Act, The 1968 Part VI. Promotion of sales of medicinal products. The Stationery Office, London

Medicines (Advertising) Amendment Regulations, The 1996 No. 1552. The Stationery Office, London

Medicines (Advertising) Regulations, The 1994 No. 1932. The Stationery Office, London

Medicines (Advertising and Monitoring of Advertising) Amendment Regulations, The 1999 No. 267.

Medicines (Monitoring of Advertising) Regulations, The 1994 No. 1933. The Stationery Office, London

Prescription Medicines Code of Practice Authority (PMCPA) 1996 The internet and the code of practice for the pharmaceutical industry. Code of Practice Review: May (PMCPA, 12 Whitehall, London, SW1A 2DY.

Telephone 020 7930 9677 Facsimile 020 7930 4554. The Code of Practice Review is published quarterly)

Prescription Medicines Code of Practice Authority (PMCPA) 1998 ABPI code of practice for the pharmaceutical industry. PMCPA, London

Proprietary Association of Great Britain (PAGB) Code of practice for advertising over-the-counter medicines to health professionals and the retail trade. PAGB, London (PAGB, Vernon House, Sicilian Avenue, London, WC1A 2QH. Telephone 0171 242 8331)

Proprietary Association of Great Britain (PAGB) Code of practice for advertising over-the-counter medicines. PAGB, London

World Health Organization (WHO) 1998 Ethical criteria for medicinal drug promotion (ISBN 92 4 154239). WHO, Geneva

Chapter 17

Legal and ethical requirements for drug information pharmacists

David Hands and Elena Grant

Introduction

In general, drug information centres in hospitals are staffed by pharmacists. In addition to being subject to legislation, employer requirements, and general ethical principles, pharmacists will also be subject to the legal and ethical principles which govern the practice of the profession of pharmacy.

In the UK the Royal Pharmaceutical Society has issued a Code of Ethics (Royal Pharmaceutical Society of Great Britain 1999*) comprising nine principles supplemented by more detailed obligations. The Code of Ethics includes guidance which is intended to help in the interpretation of the Code. Many of the principles and obligations refer to aspects of pharmacy other than drug information and will not be discussed here. Those which are relevant to the provision of drug information are discussed in this chapter.

Principles

- A pharmacist's prime concern must be for the welfare of both the patient and other members of the public.
- A pharmacist must at all times have regard to the laws and regulations applicable to pharmaceutical practice and maintain a high standard of professional conduct.
- A pharmacist must respect the confidentiality of information acquired in the course of professional practice relating to a patient and the patient's family. Such information must not be disclosed to anyone without the consent of the patient or appropriate guardian unless the interest of the patient or the public requires such disclosure.
- A pharmacist must keep abreast of the progress of pharmaceutical knowledge in order to maintain a high standard of professional competence relative to his sphere of activity.

The Code of Ethics also covers standards. Those for hospital pharmacy include the requirement that evaluated, independent information and advice on medicines will be available to all health professionals. This ensures that knowledge of medicines and their use is maximized to enhance pharmaceutical care of patients.

Apart from the legal and ethical principles which apply to the practice of pharmacy, the UK Drug Information Pharmacists Group, which coordinates drug information work, has made recommendations on those principles that are specifically relevant to drug information (Judd 1997).

*At the time of writing, the Code of Ethics is in the process of undergoing substantial revision

Liability

If an information pharmacist acting in a professional capacity provides information and/or advice to a clinician, nurse, or patient regarding, for example, the use of drugs and if this is acted on and leads to loss and/or damage to the patient, then the drug information pharmacist may be liable in negligence. The same applies to a clinician or employer, dependent on the individual circumstances. In such a case the onus would be on the pharmacist to prove that there was no negligence and that all action was in accordance with the accepted standard of care owed to the patient. The standard of care is measured against the high standards of the profession. It is assessed by asking the question, 'How would the reasonably competent pharmacist have acted in similar circumstances?'

Negligence

In order for any action in negligence to succeed against a drug information pharmacist, the plaintiff (person bringing the action) must show:

- a duty to take care was owed to him by the drug information pharmacist
- a breach of that duty
- resulting damage to the plaintiff.

The plaintiff would have to show that the defendant failed to exercise the skill and knowledge which a professional person in the same position could reasonably have been expected to have. The drug information pharmacist, as a general rule, would not be negligent if he or she acted in accordance with accepted practice at the time, as decided by a responsible body of competent professional opinion.

Drug information pharmacists have a duty to keep their professional knowledge and practice up to date. Failure to use a particular procedure or source of information that was available could be classified as negligence, if a competent and prudent pharmacist would have used that procedure or source. If a comment is made upon the information supplied and a course of action is recommended, the drug information pharmacist is substituting his/her knowledge for that of the recipient and could be regarded as negligent if the patient suffered harm due to negligent advice. Errors of judgement are to be expected and do not necessarily give rise to liability, provided reasonable care and skill have been used in reaching the judgement.

A notice disclaiming liability for the consequences of the provision of incorrect information may be included with written material. However, such a notice is ineffective in so far as it attempts to restrict liability with regard to personal injury or death sustained by a third party. In any event such notices are only effective in so far as they are fair and reasonable in the circumstances.

It is important to inform prescribers that they could be liable in law if they use unlicensed drugs and a patient is harmed and if negligence is proved. Similar liability could arise from using licensed drugs for indications or in doses outside the terms of the licence as included in the summary of product characteristics.

It is recommended that drug information pharmacists:

- ensure that the Code of Ethics and the standard of practice are officially approved by local management
- ensure that all staff working in drug information units are aware of and adhere to agreed standards of practice
- include disclaimers as advised in written material, e.g. bulletins
- ensure that the job description includes all aspects of work done

- take advice from their employers' legal advisors
- have indemnity insurance.

Provision of information for legal purposes

Drug information pharmacists may be asked to supply standard information about a drug, e.g. identification, mode of action, adverse effects etc. If a comment or opinion is provided, the drug information pharmacist would be functioning as an 'expert witness' and may have to give evidence at any resulting court hearing. Any request to attend is mandatory.

Information for coroners

It should be made clear that the pharmacist has expertise in drug information rather than in any particular aspect of applied therapeutics or medicine. As with other healthcare professionals, the drug information pharmacist may also be called as a witness of fact and/or expert witness. A coroner's summons cannot be refused.

Information supplied to the police

Information as above provided for legal purposes and for coroners applies similarly to information provided to the police. If the police request information or a comment on a patient's therapy, the confidentiality clause which binds a doctor and patient, also binds the drug information pharmacist and patient. Many National Health Service trusts have procedures relating to the release of such information, and drug information pharmacists are advised to check local procedures, and where appropriate only provide such information with permission of the trust.

Information supplied to legal representatives of patients or other persons

The advice given above also applies here. Drug information pharmacists may be approached by solicitors handling shoplifting or driving offences where the effects of drugs may be put forward as a defence. In such cases it may be preferable to provide such information to the doctor of the subject concerned, since the doctor may be best qualified to assess it in context. If information is supplied directly to legal representatives this should be done with full managerial support in line with local policies and with regard to patient confidentiality.

Active data dissemination

If an error occurs in a bulletin, abstract, new product assessment etc., the concept of negligence may apply. Should a patient suffer personal injury as a result of such an error, the author(s) could be involved in legal proceedings.

Disclaimers have been used in an attempt to avoid or minimize liability. They do not allow the author(s) to escape liability as far as the patient is concerned. They may be of use in the question of division of responsibility between, for example, prescriber and drug information pharmacist, but should not be relied upon to escape liability. The following statements are recommended:

- 'Not to be used for commercial purposes:'
- 'This bulletin has been prepared by a drug information pharmacist from standard information sources and references available at the time of publication. It may therefore need to be revised in the light of new information:'

Any recommendations by legal advisors acting for a trust or other employers should be followed.

Liability towards pharmaceutical companies in respect of statements made about their products

In preparing drug information bulletins etc., the drug information pharmacist must ensure that information contained in the bulletin are matters of fact or fair comment (i.e. expressions of opinion based on true facts). A company whose product is criticized might formulate a complaint in libel or malicious falsehood, or as defamation if the company lost sales as a result of inaccurate information or unfair comment. A simple innocent error, made in good faith and redressed by a promptly published correction, would probably not be actionable.

Drug information pharmacists should take every care to check the accuracy of any critical comments about drugs, and any agreed procedures followed.

Abstracts

Errors may arise in the production of abstracts. It is recommended that a cautionary statement on the use of abstracts is issued to users, e.g. 'Abstracts are not intended to be used as a primary source of information, but as an aid to help the searcher decide whether or not an article is relevant to a problem. The user is advised to consult the original article.'

Confidentiality of information

Information relating to patients must be regarded as confidential. Such confidentiality of information relating to a patient or guardian must normally be maintained unless in certain circumstances it is considered that the interest of the patient or the public requires such disclosure. Professional judgement should be used in assessing the risks and benefits when considering such confidentiality.

The decision to break patient confidentiality may be difficult. The following examples illustrate the point:

- A member of the public telephones to ask for information on the drug zidovudine. She has found the drug in her husband's bedside cabinet. She did not realize he was taking any drugs and wants to know what the drug is for.

In this case the husband has the right to confidentiality. It is probable, however, that the drug is being taken because he is HIV positive, and he could well be putting his wife at risk as HIV can be transmitted by sexual intercourse. There is therefore an argument that the wife has the right to the information as her health could be put at risk.

- A very agitated mother calls to ask the drug information pharmacist to identify a white tablet she has found in her 15-year-old daughter's bedroom.

In this case it is possible that the tablet is an oral contraceptive, a drug of abuse, or a tablet prescribed by a doctor or bought legally over the counter. Patient confidentiality would normally be respected, except if the pharmacist considered that it was in the patient's interests for disclosure to be made.

The identity of each enquirer should also be regarded as confidential and withheld from a third party (e.g. clinical expert or pharmaceutical company) unless specific approval is obtained from the enquirer. Similarly, certain types of information, e.g. that supplied by manufacturers regarding formulations, could be confidential and for use only for individual patient care. Such confidentiality must be respected.

The UK Data Protection Act also imposes requirements and restrictions on personal data held on computer or as manual records. Drug information pharmacists should register relevant data via the employer's data protection coordinator.

Copyright

Drug information pharmacists must also comply with copyright legislation (see Chapter 18).

References   Judd A (ed) 1997 Legal and ethical aspects of drug information. In: UK drug information manual. 4th edn. UK Drug Information Pharmacists Group, ch. 3 (available from: Drugs and Poisons Information Service, The General Infirmary, Great George Street, Leeds LS1 3EX, UK)

Royal Pharmaceutical Society of Great Britain. Medicines, Ethics and Practice 1999 A guide for pharmacists.

or identical. However, outright copying, such as photocopying the artwork of a structure diagram is infringement and should be avoided, or permission sought. It makes no difference if the chemical structure were created by some software from a 3D database.

What if someone has licensed a particular database and wants to search it using a different software from that provided?

The contract may well bundle the software with the database. Any data supplier who tried to enforce a contract that did not permit searching the database using some other software is probably open to an action for restraint of trade.

Moral rights

Moral rights are different from copyright. There are three. The first is the right for the author of a work to be acknowledged as the author or creator, the so-called paternity right. The second right, which applies whether you have ever created anything or not, is the right to object to your name being attributed to something you did not create. The third is the right not to have your work subjected to 'derogatory' treatment, that is to some amendment that impugns your integrity or reputation.

Moral rights, unlike copyrights, are not transferable and therefore always remain with the creator, even if the creator has chosen to assign his or her copyright in the material. Creators in the UK (not elsewhere) also must choose to assert the first of the moral rights, the paternity right (in other words, that right is not automatic as copyright is). It is also worth noting that in some circumstances, moral rights can never exist in UK law, for example if you are an employee who is paid to create copyright material in the course of your employment, you have no moral rights to that material. Oddly, some moral rights also do not apply to journal articles. These restrictions do not apply in other countries.

There are several ways that moral rights issues might arise in an information environment, and it is important not to trivialize or ignore the issue. An action that may be legal from a copyright point of view may nonetheless infringe moral rights. Remember, because moral rights can never be assigned, it is quite irrelevant what copyright clearances you have obtained from the copyright owner. Specifically, one should always ensure that the name of the creator or author remains associated with the work, and that material should never be quoted out of context in such a way that it gives a misleading impression of what the creator intended. Some commentators have argued that moral rights will become more important than copyright in terms of legal restraint on the use of copyright materials in the 21st century.

Liability

Liability is the duty of care that one individual or organization owes to another, and is also the risk of being sued for damages if the individual or organization fails in that duty. In the UK there is no Act of Parliament or other regulation that deals explicitly with the liability for provision of information. The three areas of UK law that potentially affect the legal liability of information provision are contract law, tort, and strict liability.

The first area of law that might apply is contract law. A contract is an agreement between two parties. One party offers to do something for the other, the other party accepts this offer. Contracts need not be in writing and signed, and it is a common misunderstanding that they must involve the exchange of money. A contract can be verbal (although, of course, it will be harder to prove there was an offer and acceptance if it was not recorded), and certainly no money need change hands for a contract to take effect. The contract obliges the parties to do certain things. Although in theory the contract can be one-sided, in practice the Unfair Contract Terms Act 1977 requires that the clauses (if any are written down) are subject to the test of reasonableness. The law also implies certain terms in any contract. In particular, a supplier of goods and services should apply reasonable skill and care in the provision of those goods or services. You are liable when you fail to fulfil your obligations under the contract, or do not exercise reasonable skill or care. Only the parties directly involved in the contract can sue for such a breach of contract.

Tort is part of case law. There is an assumption that citizens owe each other a duty of care. If you cause your fellow citizens loss by your negligence, you must pay them compensation. Tort does not require any contractual relationship between the parties involved. Therefore third parties who suffer a loss because of your actions may sue for compensation. The injured party must prove that he was owed a duty of care by the other party, that this duty was breached, there was damage, and that the damage was a direct result of the breach, and could have been reasonably foreseen. Liability depends on whether you could have reasonably foreseen that this damage could occur, and implies some proximity in your relationship (e.g. if the victim was someone who was in the library).

The European Commission has developed the concept of strict liability for the provision of goods. 'Strict liability' means that the provider of the goods or services is liable to pay for physical damage caused by those goods or services, even if the damage was not due to negligence by the provider. In 1985, the European Commission issued a directive on liability for products. This is incorporated into UK law in the Consumer Protection Act 1987. A draft directive on liability for service provision was introduced in 1990. Nothing more has happened, and it is reasonable to assume by now that the Commission has dropped the idea. Readers are urged to be aware that this issue may arise again at short notice, however.

As far as I know, there are no UK cases of information professionals being sued. There are two cases, one German, one French, involving information providers (print publishers). They are relevant because library and information science (LIS) professionals could pass on information from these sources to their patrons, and be caught up in the liability chain. The German case involved a medical book in which a decimal point was missing from a drug dosage. Instead of a '2.5 % NaCl infusion', the text read a '25% NaCl infusion.' The publisher of the book was sued by the insurance company of the victim who received the incorrect dosage and nearly died. The insurance company of the hospital where the patient had been treated paid compensation to the patient, then sued the publisher for partial compensation saying that the publisher was partly to blame. The court found that there can never be a complete absence of misprints in a print product. Publishers of specialist products, such as medical texts, should make all efforts to avoid these misprints and could be held responsible for the mistakes of proofreaders and authors. However, in this case, every medically educated person should have noticed the misprint, since the particular infusion is a common treatment. Therefore the hospital's compensation claim was rejected.

The important conclusion from this case is that if the recipient of the information is a professional, the liability for information provision is somewhat reduced as the recipient can be expected to use his or her own judgement on the validity of the information received.

In the second case, a practical guide to edible fruits and plants that was published in Germany was translated into French and published in France. The guide described the wild carrot as being edible. Someone confused the wild carrot with hemlock, which is very similar, but poisonous. This person died as a result. The court held the publishers of the book in Germany and France liable because the publishers had a duty to make sure that readers could rely on the contents of a book on edible plants and fruits. They should have verified the accuracy of information in the book before distributing it. The German author was also held to be negligent.

The key point here was that the information was passed to members of the general public, who could not be expected to use professional judgement on the quality of the information.

Chapter 19

Career development in pharmaceutical information management

Sharon Leighton

Introduction

Working in the pharmaceutical industry or related healthcare services presents particular challenges for information professionals. Knowledge about medicines, clinical practice, health technology, biomedical sciences, molecular biology and chemistry continues to boom, with increasingly diverse sources and knowledge management systems to consult. A variety of professional roles exists to effectively exploit and manage this information. This chapter will explore the skills, competencies and qualities required of information professionals. Let us start by looking at the range of functions within information management in the pharmaceutical industry.

Information careers in the pharmaceutical industry

The pharmaceutical industry offers exciting opportunities for information professionals, depending upon their science background and personal interests. The flow of information and management of knowledge are critical at all areas and levels within the organization, ranging from the initial drug discovery through to drug development and product launch and finally to post-marketing support. For companies to become and stay successful, they increasingly need to develop better drugs more quickly and more new chemical entities per year. Information and knowledge about potential new therapies and disease processes are vital to making sound business decisions. Pharmaceutical information management is therefore a core value-added business process.

Roles of information professionals in research & development (R&D)

During the drug discovery phase, chemists, pharmacologists, geneticists, biochemists and toxicologists work together in partnerships with research information professionals. Typically, the role of these information professionals is to identify new developments of interest and recently published work, maintain scientific records and provide the tools and training for the scientists to become more information aware themselves. End-user searching has often been seen as a threat to research information professionals. Yet the deluge of information available in a wider diversity of media has emphasized the need for the skills of information professionals to research, filter and analyse material to help the drug discoverers gain knowledge and insight.

Bioinformatics is a developing specialization within the industry. Professionals involved in this area may analyse DNA sequences from a wide range of sources to fit the research project requirements. On a more proactive basis they also provide DNA sequence information to drug discovery scientists using data mining techniques.

As promising drug compounds progress through the stages of development into products, different specialist skills are required. The customer group shifts more towards applied science in areas such as toxicology, clinical pharmacology, regulatory affairs, pharmaceutical development, drug safety and pre-launch marketing.

Records management is critical at all these stages to ensure that the company conforms to the standards of Good Laboratory Practice and Good Clinical Practice. Professional librarians play a key role. They use a wide range of sources to provide high quality information, tailored to a customer's exact needs (Library Association 1995).

Role of information professionals in the commercial marketing organization

During the later stages of development of a product, the commercial operations in the company become increasingly involved in its launch and then its post-marketing development. The focus turns to the business and medical information professionals. Business information staff tend to have prior commercial experience (for example, as sales representatives) which helps them understand their key customers—marketing and sales personnel. They track sales and competitor performance using in-house and commercial databases, predicting trends and future business performance.

Medical information is a well-developed profession within the industry in the UK. Dealing with customer enquiries usually forms the larger part of the day-to-day work. This role presents its own challenges due to the diverse customer base and wide-ranging enquiry types. The regular contact that medical information staff have with external customers provides valuable opportunities for feedback on product issues. Careers in medical information have also been covered by Janet Taylor (1994).

On a more proactive basis, medical information staff may provide current product and competitor literature to a wide range of internal customers (e.g. marketing, medical, regulatory and sales personnel). In addition to alerting services, their role may include deeper analysis of the clinical evidence base for the company's products, competitors and their place in therapy. Other roles may include checking of promotional material for accuracy, balance and comprehensiveness, preparing prescribing information (e.g. patient information leaflets), maintaining literature databases and supporting end-user training.

The medical information role is particularly strong within the UK. In other European countries the role may be split across several groups. For example, customer enquiries may be dealt with by medically qualified staff or pharmacists whose major role is medico-marketing or regulatory affairs. Documentalists or medical librarians support their information needs. In the US, various approaches are used. Call centres using triage methods, sophisticated information and telephony systems are able to deal with enormous volumes of customer enquiries. These call centres may incorporate similar specialist information analysts and medical or pharmaceutical advisors to support the core function.

Secretarial support staff perform an important role in any information department. As well as the more traditional secretarial activities, they may be involved in many administrative tasks. Examples include maintaining chemical compound control systems, database entry, library transactions, dealing with simple enquiries (leaflet or sample requests) etc.

At a higher level, there are information managers and directors within the industry, implementing company strategy and directing the work of the teams that report to them. The role of the information manager is extensively covered in Chapter 7.

Starting out in pharmaceutical information management

The starting point when deciding if a career in pharmaceutical information management is for you is to try answering the following questions:

- Do I have the right qualifications (degree subject, degree level or further degree)?
- Do I have at least some of the right skills, competencies and qualities (see below)?
- Do any of the jobs described below sound exciting or interesting to me?
- Do I have any ethical objections to working within the pharmaceutical industry?
- Do I have any ultimate career goals in mind that would suggest alternative industry positions? For example, working as a sales representative may be regarded as more suitable experience for a future in marketing.
- Do I know anyone already working in these roles who can tell me more about what the job entails, including any positive or negative aspects?

New graduates will already have had some careers advice from their university or they may have used excellent reference sources such as *What Colour is Your Parachute* (Bolles 1998). Due to lack of experience in this field, unfortunately, few careers advisory services mention pharmaceutical information management as a career move. Many of the entrants straight from university (either post degree or post doctorate) tend to enter the industry from answering job advertisements.

Once you are convinced that information work is for you, how do you set about finding a position? Scanning job advertisements is the first step. In the UK one of the most suitable journals for placing advertisements for information management positions in the pharmaceutical industry is the *New Scientist*. Specialist journals and trade newsletters are the next choice. Examples are the *Pharmaceutical Journal* for drug information and medical information posts or *AIOPI News* (Association of Information Officers in the Pharmaceutical Industry).

Increasingly, posts can be found on the world wide web. For example, two sites, InPharm and Pharmiweb, advertise a wide range of posts in the pharmaceutical industry at all levels. Companies may advertise directly onto their websites. The Drug Information Association (DIA – http://www.diahome.org/) also advertises vacancies. It is particularly valuable for finding positions in the USA, but it covers other countries too.

On a more proactive front, it is worth writing to the human resources or personnel departments of pharmaceutical companies that you are particularly interested in. Alternatively, you can write to the information manager direct. Lists of companies in the UK can be obtained from the ABPI (Association of the British Pharmaceutical Industry) or its website (www.abpi.org.uk). As with any job application it is worth doing some background research on the company so that you can tailor your application to the company profile.

There are also a number of recruitment agencies that deal with information vacancies. Lists of recruitment agencies are available in the Flexipages section of the InPharm website (1999) or on the Pharmiweb website (1999).

Key skills for information professionals

Just as biomedical information does not stand still, neither does our need to develop our own skills and those of our staff. But just what skills, competencies and qualities are required for information professionals? How can they best acquire them?

A checklist of key skills of information professionals is useful when recruiting staff or producing a development plan. What differentiates the essential, the useful and the 'nice to have' skills and qualities? These will, of course, vary according to the type and level of the job.

Those essential skills that are core to most pharmaceutical industry information posts would include:

- a good pharmacy or science degree or further degree (e.g. MSc, PhD) along with expanding product and therapeutic specialist knowledge
- computer literacy (e.g. word processing, electronic diaries, e-mail, presentation programs and spreadsheets)
- communication skills including good oral and written skills
- interpersonal skills encompassing the basics of customer service, problem solving, time management and organizational skills.

Although skills can be taught, if necessary, most graduates should have at least basic aptitude in the above areas. Training courses cannot easily substitute for a lack of biomedical knowledge.

Other useful skills are:

- online database and internet searching
- document presentation skills
- formal presentation skills
- telephone skills
- influencing skills
- project management.

Although it is helpful if information professionals or potential recruits have these skills, they can often be taught on basic training courses.

Previous pharmaceutical industry experience is also useful as it gives information professionals a fundamental understanding of the drug development process. This makes it much easier to relate to internal customer needs as well as understand the generation of data, information and knowledge within the organization.

As personnel progress within their career, skills for further development would typically involve:

- advanced communication skills (e.g. assertiveness and negotiating skills, giving and receiving feedback, briefing and debriefing, running successful meetings, videoconferencing, net meetings)
- training others
- planning
- supervisory or managerial skills (recruitment, team building and team working, staff development, delegation, mentoring)
- understanding finance and financial control
- understanding how organizations work
- business skills.

Self and personnel development will be discussed later in this chapter.

Key qualities in information professionals

Personality characteristics are often based upon values and beliefs that develop during our early life and upbringing and so they are more difficult to influence and alter. Therefore it is worth investing in time to properly select personnel for information posts and conversely for graduates considering an information career to question whether they have the right qualities for the job.

Once more, the qualities that we look for in information professionals will depend upon the current position that they hold and level of advancement. Some useful core qualities of information professionals include:

- friendly or approachable nature
- methodical approach and attention to detail
- flexibility
- proactivity
- ability to cope under pressure
- commitment
- integrity
- confidence
- an altruistic willingness to help others.

Since information professionals invariably work closely with customers, a friendly nature with a willingness to help others (altruism) is an essential. As our work is varied, with shifting priorities, an ability to work under pressure and constantly prioritize and re-prioritize is also a necessity.

Not only is it essential to have up-to-date knowledge through our research and knowledge collections, but also to communicate that knowledge confidently in a variety of communication media (telephone conversations, e-mail, formal reports or business letters, customer presentations, training courses etc.). Without that added confidence and professionalism, our customers may lose faith in the knowledge we have to impart.

When providing information about a subject, it is important to ensure that it is balanced and that it reflects the available evidence. This responsibility requires qualities of integrity and a methodical nature.

As information professionals progress within their organizations, which are increasingly organized in flatter hierarchies, useful qualities for more senior positions include:

- credibility
- diplomacy
- approachability
- maturity
- responsibility
- awareness of culture
- initiative
- ability to network with others
- creativity and innovation
- leadership skills.

The importance of these qualities is just as great as it is for other managerial posts within the pharmaceutical industry, other 'high tech' industries and in health services. This area is discussed in more depth in the chapter on professional and managerial skills (Chapter 7).

Career progression for the pharmaceutical information professional

Career progression is a natural desire for any worker today. However, with leaner organizations and flatter organizational structures, promotion opportunities have gradually become more restricted. So just what career pathways are there in pharmaceutical information management?

There are effectively two pathways—progressing within information management or using the marketable skills that any information professional inevitably develops during his /her career.

Staying within information management

Most information professionals starting out in their career might reasonably expect to progress by moving up. However, they can also develop their careers by moving sideways, positioning themselves for moving up at a later date.

In general, job grades may progress in the following manner: from an assistant grade to an officer (executive, scientist, analyst or title used by the company), then to a senior and possibly principal position. With progression there are inevitably increasing responsibilities. There will also be expectations of greater expertise in information management and usually therapeutic area expertise and knowledge. A manager's position is one that some junior staff aspire to, although supervisory responsibility may become a feature of the senior or principal positions. A management position is not always the only choice when progressing within the organization. Technical or product specialization is an alternative route whereby specialist expertise and knowledge are rewarded without having to assume management responsibility.

Sideways moves within information management are an excellent way to broaden out experience, refocus a career or develop new skills. The skills acquired are likely to be relevant to many aspects of information management.

Speaking personally, I moved from neuropharmacology research at Glaxo Group Research to an information management career in cardiovascular research information. Shortly afterwards, an opportunity arose to move into the information systems group in the same organization. This job involved product information database administration and training as well as research database management. My next move was to change companies and career directions to set up and develop a medical information department.

This broad base of experience has enabled me to gain knowledge of all aspects of drug discovery, development and portfolio management. It has also given me a wide range of experience in many aspects of information management, including online searching, end-user training, database design and administration, setting up new services, team recruitment and management, and global networking. I have also gained considerable business awareness.

Changing the type of organization that you work for can also provide an opportunity for career progression. Working for a larger or a smaller organization can give you different experience. If you currently work within a large department but would like to have more direct influence or create more opportunities to broaden your experience, working for a smaller organization can bring a new lease of life.

New ways of working

Organizations are increasingly changing the ways in which they operate and organize their workforce. Charles Handy has extensively discussed this change in several of his books. In *The Age of Unreason*, he describes the Shamrock Organization, which has reorganized its workforce to provide greater flexibility with reduced costs (Handy 1995). The organization employs three types of workers:

- full-time knowledge workers with specialized expertise
- part-time, hourly or temporary workers who are flexible and provide less complex skills
- contract workers who also possess specialized expertise provided on a consulting or contract basis.

The full range in a pharmaceutical company might include full-time employees working on site, teleworkers, part-timers, job shares and contractors as well as some functions that are completely outsourced to other service industries. This trend has been determined by organizational change as well as people's response to changing work patterns. As jobs have become more demanding, some professionals have re-evaluated their career and considered 'downshifting'. Although this may imply a demotion or have negative connotations, it can be a very positive step for some people. The gains achieved are usually enhancements in lifestyle.

Where do we see these alternative work styles within information management? Certain functions can be outsourced or run using alternative work patterns. Examples include manning help desks or hotlines. Some smaller companies outsource enquiries on minor products or products with specific patient information needs to external agencies.

Working within information management provides us with the opportunity to develop transportable skills. In turn, this provides us with more career choice, allowing us to consider alternative work patterns yet still gain job satisfaction and financial security.

In his book *The Empty Raincoat*, Charles Handy (1994) develops the theme of changing work patterns. He uses the term 'going portfolio' to describe doing a variety of different jobs to satisfy our different needs. However we may only receive pay for part of the work that we do.

Many information professionals working within the pharmaceutical industry and in health services are young women—over three-quarters of the membership of AIOPI are female. Some will start a family at some point in their career, which brings a whole realm of new pressures but also choices. Being realistic, women still tend to bear the responsibility for organizing childcare and household management. The demands of juggling family needs and a full-time career are extremely high and that is not the lifestyle choice for all. Therefore a certain proportion choose to refocus their career and work in more flexible ways.

Within pharmaceutical information management, there are a number of people (mainly women) who work part-time. This can sometimes be as a permanent staff member (depending upon company policy), as a job share with a colleague or working as an agency contractor. In these examples, staff usually work on site for at least part of the time to fulfil their responsibilities. Alternatively, there are some tasks that can be done by staff working from home, as independent consultants or teleworking. If this is an option that you wish to consider and want to know more, there are a number of general publications or websites that discuss working from home, teleworking or freelancing (Gil Gordon website, Glenny & Mullinger 1997, Nash 1999).

Moving on

The skills and experience that we develop as information professionals make us extremely marketable. This gives us opportunities to use these skills in other areas such as:

- information technology, information services
- pharmacovigilance
- clinical research
- medical writing
- marketing (although previous sales experience is often required)
- regulatory affairs
- business information.

Looking outside the pharmaceutical industry, some staff progress into positions with information management suppliers (e.g. database producers or hosts, information systems and software, publishing, medical communications etc.). As the pharmaceutical industry is regarded as a good employer compared with many other industries, many people stay on.

Self-development for the information professional

Managing our self-development is a major responsibility of every information professional, regardless of skill level. Equally, information managers need to develop their staff as well as their own skills. Development is essential for furthering our careers, for acquiring new skills, for growing our skills further and to improve our competencies and abilities.

Although the organizations that we work for may play a role in improving our skills and help us determine the pathway that we take, this is not always the case. Managers may fail to develop themselves or their staff because they may think that they do not have the time to devote to it. They may not appreciate the importance of self-development, they may not have the knowledge or they may be worried about staff progressing further than them. A common misunderstanding is that there is not sufficient budget for training courses and so it is not worth considering staff training or development. As will become apparent, staff or self-development does not just mean attending training courses—it can be implemented using other imaginative methods.

The benefits of developing ourselves are many. Personally, we need different skills and qualities for different roles and for career progression. From an organizational standpoint, staff development is essential to retain high-quality personnel, thus reducing recruitment and staff induction costs and improving return on training investment. Self-development is motivational for most people; self-actualization is one of the most important driving factors of human beings.

If management is about achieving results through people, then people can be developed by involvement in tasks and projects which provide a challenge for them. Staff development is also investment for the future. The pace of change within organizations now means that we need to be better prepared to face challenges as they arise. Staff must be prepared to take on more demanding work. Charles Handy (1994) quotes '1/2 × 2 × 3 = P' as the policy of a chairman of a pharmaceutical company in his book, *The Empty Raincoat*. This formula translates as half the number of people working for the company paid twice as well for doing three times the amount of work equals profit. When we move towards this situation, highly skilled people are essential.

How do we determine which skills we need to develop? There are many tools to help us pinpoint which areas we need to focus upon, identify the gap and thus the training need. At its simplest, we can match our current skill breadth and depth against our job descriptions. At its most complex, we can be independently assessed at a self-assessment centre or through professional career counselling. Other methods could include SWOT analyses, where we assess our strengths and weaknesses, the opportunities and the possible threats.

Training departments, libraries and professional organizations can provide materials, advice or support. A number of books can help—a visit to a good bookshop will probably be all that you need to find a book that suits you. Alternatively see References and further reading for some suggestions.

When we have a clearer picture of the areas where we need to develop, we should set the aims and objectives of our development plan and then consider which methods to use. When setting objectives for ourselves or for our staff, they need to be challenging but achievable. For example, if we are using a project as a development tool, we have to monitor the situation to ensure that the project can be completed successfully without causing too much stress to the person concerned. We need to remember that we/they are not only doing the project, we/they also need time to learn new skills or further grow existing skills.

Once we are clear about what we want to achieve in our own development or that of our staff, we need to consider different training methods. There are a wide variety that we can use, suitable for differing situations and needs. Although everyone immediately thinks 'training course' when he or she considers self-development, this may often be the least effective route unless properly thought through and implemented and progress is monitored.

What other methods can we use? Examples include:

- On the job training by the manager. As this is often at the initial stage in a job, it is important that it is structured, using a set plan, that progress is regularly monitored and skilled coaching techniques are used.
- Appropriate reading or distance learning if available. Within our own field, material from journals or industry magazines is helpful, and this book is intended to act as a source in this area.
- Work shadowing. This can be suitable for someone first starting out using the technique of 'see what I do, then try it yourself'. It is also excellent for assessing a career change or refocus.
- Job secondment or job rotation. Some personnel enter into information management from other routes, seconded from another area. Examples include a sales representative moving into medical information, bench scientist into research information etc. This can add to a team's strength, since recruitment is from a prime customer group and the new recruit can provide an external, fresh look at the services and processes.

- Job enhancement by adding additional responsibilities or dealing with key customers.
- Project work, as long as it is a meaningful project with appropriate level of support from the manager.
- Promotion.
- Work on special interest groups. Examples in the UK include professional bodies such as AIOPI, the Institute of Information Scientists, Aslib and, outside the UK, the Drug Information Association. Involvement in such groups is an excellent way to develop a wide variety of skills (Coult 1999).
- Delegating various tasks or responsibilities (suitable for managers developing their team members).
- Training courses. There are a variety of courses and training opportunities relevant to particular therapeutic areas, or in information management or interpersonal skills training. Courses are advertised on the internet as well as through direct mail or trade journals. To be worthwhile, there needs to be a clear brief or objective agreed with the attendee and structured follow-up and monitoring of performance.
- Further qualifications. Various university courses are available that are relevant to information professionals. They include postgraduate courses in information science, management studies and other subjects, and the diploma/MSc course in Pharmaceutical Information Management at London's City University.

Using the various methods, in the right context, we have the tools at our hands to reach our true potential.

References

Bolles R N 1998 What colour is your parachute? 1999 A practical manual for job hunters & career changers. Ten Speed Press, London

Coult G 1999 Get a life! Become active in a special interest group. Managing Information 6(3): 20–21

Glenny H, Mullinger B 1998 The ACRPI guide to freelancing. ACRPI, Maidenhead

Handy C 1994 The empty raincoat. Making sense of the future. Arrow Books, London

Handy C 1995 The age of unreason. Arrow Books, London

InPharm website address: www.inpharm.com. Accessed on 1st June 1999. Webmaster Peter Llewelwyn.

Library Association 1995 Professional librarians. A brief guide for employers. Professional Practice Series

Nash S 1999 Becoming a consultant. How to start and run a profitable consulting business. How to Books, Oxford

Peel M 1989 Developing our staff. Aslib Proceedings 41(10) 301–309

Pharmiweb website address: www.pharmiweb.com. Accessed on 14th May 1999.

Taylor J 1994 Careers in Medical Information. In: Stonier P D (ed) Discovering new medicines: Careers in pharmaceutical research and development. John Wiley, Chichester

Teleworking websites:

www.gilgordon.com. Accessed 28th April. 1999. Gil Gordon Associates.

www.eto.org.uk. Accessed 28th April 1999. European Telework Online.

www.tca.org.uk. Accessed 28th April 1999. The Telework, Telecottage And Telecentre Association.

Further Reading

Mulligan J 1988 The personal management handbook. How to make the most of your potential. Sphere Reference, London

Pedler M, Burgoyne J, Boydell T 1994 A managers guide to self-development, 3rd edn. McGraw-Hill, London

Glossary

ABPI   The Association of the British Pharmaceutical Industry.

ADME   Absorption, Distribution, Metabolism, Excretion.

Adverse drug reaction (ADR)   An ADR is an adverse event associated with the use of medication.

Adverse event (AE)   Any undesirable experience occurring to a patient treated with a pharmaceutical product whether or not considered drug-related. An AE is synonymous with adverse experience.

AIOPI   The UK Association of Information Officers in the Pharmaceutical Industry.

Benefit   Is the probability that the patient benefits from the medication.

Causality   Assesses the likelihood that the suspected drug caused the AE in an individual case.

CD-ROM   Compact Disk-Read Only Memory

Client-server   A network architecture in which processing is shared by workstations (clients) and a server. Typically the workstation handles the setting up of requests and the display of data and the server processes the requests.

Clinical Trial Exemption (CTX)   CTX is the licence for clinical trials issued by the MCA in the UK. In the past, there was also a Clinical Trial Application (CTA).

CMR   Centre for Medicines Research.

Desktop computer   See PC.

DIA   The US Drug Information Association.

DMPK   Drug Metabolism and Pharmacokinetics.

Domain name   A domain is a group of computers or devices on a network that are administered as a single unit. On the Internet, each domain has a unique domain name, e.g. aiopi.org.uk. Domain names are used in URLs to locate web pages, for example: http://www.aiopi.org.uk/index.htm and in email addresses.

EHR   Electronic health record. Term used by the UK Department of Health to describe the concept of a longitudinal record of patient's health and healthcare from cradle to grave.

EPAR   European Public Assessment Report. A document issued for a medicine that has received a Marketing Authorization through the European Medicines Evaluation Agency. It provides a summary of the information submitted to the Agency about the product, including efficacy and safety data.

EPR   Electronic patient record. Term used by the UK Department of Health to describe a record containing a patient's personal details, their diagnosis or condition, and details about the treatment/assessments undertaken by a clinician.

Food and Drug Administration (FDA)   FDA is the US regulatory authority.

FTP   File transfer protocol. The network protocol used for transferring binary data files from one computer to another over the internet.

GCP   Good Clinical Practice

GLP   Good Laboratory Practice

GMP   Good Manufacturing Practice

Genetic profile   Is a tool for understanding an individual's susceptibility to medical disorders.

Gopher   Probably the most popular of the text-searching tools for locating information on the Internet prior to the advent of the worldwide web, but now almost totally superseded by the WWW.

Groupware Computer software designed to facilitate multiple users sharing work over a computer network, often working in locations remote from each other.

GUI Graphical user interface. A program interface that uses the computer's graphics capabilities to make the program easier to use by freeing the user from learning complex command languages. The key features are a pointer, a pointing device such as a mouse and a desktop containing windows, icons and pull-down menus. Microsoft Windows and web browsers are examples.

Higher Level Group Term (HLGT) In classification systems for terms used in pharmacovigilance HLGTs classify groups of HLTs.

Higher Level Term (HLT) HLTs classify groups of preferred terms (PTs).

ICH International Conference on Harmonization.

IMPI The UK association of Information Managers in the Pharmaceutical Industry.

Information classification

Investigational New Drug (IND) IND licence is required for clinical trials by the FDA, analogous to CTX.

Knowledgebase A centralized database with searchable archive of information, to which users can add their own observations and experiences.

Labelled Expected ADR. See unexpectedness.

LAN Local area network. This is a computer network which is restricted to a single site.

Listed Those ADRs listed in the core SPC.

Medicines Control Agency (MCA) MCA is the UK regulatory authority.

Metadata Data about data. In a document database, for example, the documents are the data and keyword fields such as title, author and input date are the metadata.

NCE New Chemical Entity.

NDA New Drug Application.

Network A collection of computers, storage devices and output devices that are connected to each other for the transfer of data. See also LAN and WAN.

NME New Molecular Entity.

PC Personal computer, a self-contained computer in which the main processor is located within a computer case which is connected directly to a keyboard and visual display unit.

PDF Portable document format. A proprietary document image format developed by the Adobe Corporation, which is widely used for document interchange as web browsers can be configured to read PDF files.

PDR The European Pharma Documentation Ring.

Pharmacogenetics Is the study of genetic variability and its effect on response to drug therapy.

Pharmacovigilance All methods of assessment and prevention of adverse drug reactions. The framework of pharmacovigilance is broader than that of post-marketing surveillance and includes clinical and even pre-clinical development of drugs.

Preferred Term (PT) In classification systems for terms used in pharmacovigilance, a PT classifies a group of included terms that may be synonymous or equivalent in other ways.

R&D Research and Development.

Relatedness In the context of an adverse experience in a patient receiving a drug, relatedness means a reasonable possibility that the experience may have been caused by the drug (FDA 1998).

Retention scheduling

Retention time

Risk The probability that something will happen.

SAR Structure-activity relationships.

Side-effect AAny unintended effect of medication related to the pharmacological properties of the drug.

Signal Information that an AE may be drug-related.

SOP Standard Operating Procedure.

Strict liability Defective products are liable without the need to prove negligence.

Summary of Product Characteristics (SPC)   In the European Union the SPC is a document that provides information about the composition, indications, dosage, side-effects and other information about a medicine.

System Organ Class (SOC)   SOC is often used as the top level of medical classification and has some equivalence of meaning with body system.

TCP/IP   Transmission control protocol/internet protocol. The communication protocol adopted for the internet and other information management tools which provides a common standard for transfer of data between a wide range of platforms and operating systems.

Telemedicine   A healthcare related activity involving a professional and a patient (or one professional and another) who are separated in space, facilitated by the use of information technology.

Terminal   A form of computer workstation which has no processor of its own but consists only of a keyboard and visual display unit which are connected to a central computer.

Teratogenesis   Adverse drug effects on the fetus during early pregnancy.

Unexpectedness   Occurrence of an AE that is inconsistent with ADR defined in the appropriate text such as Summary of Product. Characteristics (SPC) or the investigator brochure for Investigational New Drugs (IND).

URL   Uniform resource locator. A unique name for each page on the WWW or within an intranet consisting of the domain name, an optional directory or folder name and a filename, and prefixed by the Internet protocol appropriate for the file (http or ftp), e.g. http://www.aiopi.org.uk/articles/apr98_01.htm. Web browsers will assume the http prefix if a prefix is omitted.

WAN   Wide area network. This is a computer network that links different physical sites into a single private network.

Worldwide web (WWW)   A vast collection of documents on the Internet which are all viewable by a standard GUI interface (web browser) and named in such a way that jumping (hyperlinking) from one to another is easy. The WWW was responsible for the rapid explosion in popularity of the internet as access to data had previously required the use of text-based searching tools such as Gopher.

WORM   A non-rewritable optical disk for mass storage of computer files. Short for 'write once, read many times'.

XML   Extensible markup language. A new version of markup language which enables information to be stored in text files in a structured fashion. XML files require separate stylesheets to determine how the information will be displayed.

Index

Note: page numbers in **bold** are major topics (chapters) and those in *italics* are glossary definitions. References are to *information* and *United Kingdom*, except where otherwise indicated.